NATIVE AMERICAN HERBALIST MASTERY

6 BOOKS IN 1

The Ultimate Ancient Herbal Remedies Encyclopedia to
Create Your Natural Homemade Apothecary with Original
Dispensatory Recipes for a Lifelong Wellness

ENOLA HILL

TABLE OF CONTENTS

BOOK 1
HISTORY AND INTRODUCTION
TO HERBALISM

CHAPTER ONE: THE HISTORY OF NATIVE AMERICAN MEDICINE

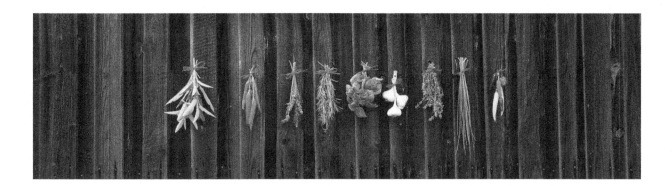

The Native Americans did not have advanced science like we do today so they had to rely solely on the native herbs in their region for the treatment of ailments. In order to know which herbs to use and what poisonous plants to avoid, the Native Americans observed sick animals and took note of the particular herbs they ate and how quickly they recovered after feeding on those herbs. This led to the discovery of various medicinal plants that were used in treating ailments in humans. Some of these plants are sage, cedar, sweetgrass, and tobacco plants. These four were considered sacred and together with other local herbs, they were used to treat their diseases.

The Native Americans had what they called the medicine wheel. The medicine wheel was used to create a balance with nature which the people believed was necessary to the human body for total and holistic healing. This balance was required because the indigenous people believed in curing the source of the problem instead of just taking away the symptoms. They believed that most illnesses had spiritual connections; hence, they focused on creating a balance between the spiritual and the physical in healing diseases.

They also had their medicine men that took care of the plants, made sure medicinal herbs were always readily available, and knew exactly what each plant cured. The medicine men were highly revered in Native America as their jobs were considered even sacred. The medicine men were also spiritualists who could use incense and some spiritual ceremonies to purify the atmosphere.

Native Americans used different kinds of herbs to heal diseases. These include the white palm, wild yam, sage plant, and cedar. The sage, cedar, sweetgrass, and tobacco were considered the four sacred plants by the indigenous people. Some of the other ingredients used by Native Americans for ailments include wild yam, white pine, and slippery elm. The native healing style usually includes the burning of objects, storytelling, herbs, and music.

The Native Americans also did minor surgeries. They made syringes out of hollow bones with which they performed their surgeries. They were orthopedics and extremely good at bone massages. Their surgeries were even better and more humane than the early European surgeries due to the fact that the natives made use of natural anesthesia for surgical procedures.

The Native American medicine bag was famously used for storing herbs and other medicinal items and was believed to give power to its owner. Some of the bag's contents were the four sacred items; that is, cedar, sage, sweetgrass, and tobacco. The medicine man also had other medicinal items in the bag, but the sage, tobacco, cedar, and sweetgrass were deemed the most important.

We have mentioned the sage plant a few times for its medicinal powers, but we are yet to talk about the reason the sage was considered sacred. The sage was considered sacred because, apart from being used for its medicinal purposes, it can be used to cleanse an environment of bad spirits, purify people's homes and bring about mental calm. The white sage was primarily used to fortify the venues during ceremonies which allow the passage of good spirits and repulsion of bad ones. The white sage plant has a unique smoke that is believed to create a barrier that prevents evil spirits from entering certain ceremonies.

The sage plant has antifungal, antiseptic, and anti-inflammatory properties. It is a natural antioxidant that protects the human body from harmful toxins, which is the reason the sage plant is highly revered in Native American history.

It is true that most of our modern medication was first made using plants that the indigenous people have used to cure the same diseases for hundreds of years.

Some of these plants are described below.

Plants Used By Indigenous People

1. Cascara Sagrada

The Native Americans primarily used this plant as a laxative. Cascara contains chemicals known as anthraquinones. This chemical gives cascara the laxative effect that it has on the human body. Cascara is also called a stimulant laxative because it cures constipation by stimulating the muscles in the bowels. Cascara usually takes about 8 to 12 hours to work after the dosage has been taken.

As one of the oldest medications for constipation, cascara can also be taken as a dietary supplement. It can be taken as a tea or a cold drink for constipation. Although cascara is generally safe for aged people, care should be taken when taking it alongside other medication especially medication for inflammation because adding them to cascara may lower potassium levels in the body.

Though cascara is generally safe, it may pose a health challenge to some people so it is advisable to speak with a doctor before using the herb. It is important for pregnant women, nursing mothers and little children to consult physicians before taking cascada because it is not safe during pregnancy or breastfeeding.

Long term use of this herb is also discouraged because it may lead to liver damage, electrolyte imbalance, headache and reduction in urine. To make cascara tea, put a cup of water in a kettle and boil. Then add one teaspoon of cascara in the water and boil for five minutes. Allow it steep for five more minutes. Strain and drink.

2. Ginseng

The American ginseng is a medicinal plant native to North America. This plant has been used by Native Americans for many years as a medicinal herb. Ginseng has antioxidants, anti-inflammatory and antibacterial properties. These properties make ginseng an invaluable herb even in this era of modern medicine. Ginseng has a lot of medicinal benefits. Its roots are said to boost energy, lower blood sugar levels and stabilize cholesterol levels.

Ginseng is also good for the brain as it enhances brain power, keeps people alert and fights fatigue. As a result of its ability to reduce blood sugar content, it is best to take ginseng just before meals or immediately after meals in order for it to work on the sugar in the meals. Apart from blood sugar, ginseng is widely celebrated for helping with erectile dysfunction. Some people say they prefer taking natural ginseng to laboratory produced Viagra. Ginseng is better than Viagra in the sense that it is natural and has minimal side effects. It relaxes the muscles and allows free flow of blood to the genitals.

Ginseng has been proved to improve sexual function for men with erectile dysfunction. Ginseng is also good for fighting different kinds of cancer. Panax ginseng is known for improving sexual function for men however, it should be used on a shorter basis as long-term use may cause side effects. Furthermore, ginseng helps with moods because it calms the nerves and minimizes feelings of depression. Ginseng also boosts metabolism which results in weight loss.

In addition to all these benefits, ginseng increases breast and buttocks sizes. It does this by triggering the endocrine glands which simulate the production of estrogen. When used to prevent an illness, ginseng effectively reduces the duration of the disease. It should be noted that ginseng should not be used for more than two months at a time as prolonged use can cause some side effects.

3. Garlic

Garlic is one of the most recognized medicinal herbs in modern medicine. Garlic comes with a whole lot of health benefits like protecting the heart, normalizing blood pressure and reducing sugar levels in the body. Garlic extract is constantly being used to make numerous medications for humans. Garlic in its raw state has been used to treat different ailments such as high blood pressure. Garlic is effective for lowering blood pressure and cholesterol. It also allows free flow of blood to the heart which prevents heart attacks.

In addition, it cures the common cold, flu, allows for stronger bones, better memory etc. As a potent antibiotic, garlic is an effective treatment for yeast infection like Candida. It can be taken orally or applied topically for yeast infection. Garlic is also good for prostate cancer as it contains properties that slows the progression of cancer cells. It can either prevent these cells from growing or slow down their growth rate.

Garlic is also potent for uterine tract infections and ear problems due to its antibiotic properties. To get rid of ear pain, put grated garlic in coconut oil or olive oil for 24 hours, warm the oil and strain. Then put this oil in the ear like you would with ear drop.

In order to achieve best results from garlic, take garlic in the morning on an empty stomach. It should be eaten raw because raw garlic has a property called allicin. Allicin regulates cholesterol levels in the body by thinning blood in the vessels. Cooked garlic does not contain allicin because heat kills that compound.

Garlic is an antiseptic, antibacterial and antifungal agent so it helps the body destroy infections. This means that garlic also acts as an immune system booster. This herb, apart from curing a lot of infections, can also help a person sleep at night because of its zinc and sulphurous compounds which allows for relaxation. The best time to eat garlic is on an empty stomach at least thirty minutes before breakfast because that is when it is most potent as the body processes only the garlic which allows the antibiotic content of garlic to fully come out and heal the body. Garlic can be taken for weight loss, vaginal yeast and stomach cancer. Simply grate 5 cloves of garlic, add to two glasses of water and drink. To make garlic tea, grate 5 cloves of garlic, add to boiling water and boil for five minutes. Let it steep for five extra minutes. Strain and drink.

Garlic also works as an appetite suppressant which means if you drink garlic tea before meals, you get to eat less but feel full for longer. To crown it all, garlic water detoxifies the body because garlic has antioxidants which flush out harmful toxins, free radicals, cancer and other infections from the body.

4. Ginkgo

Ginkgo is a medicinal plant native to the Northern Hemisphere. This herb is used not just for its flavor but for its medicinal properties. For instance, ginkgo increases blood flow to the brain, helps with memory and improves other brain related health conditions. Ginkgo improves memory in people with Alzheimer's disease, dementia and other brain diseases. It successfully slows down the disease and also opens clogged arteries. It also helps with psychological problems like depression and ADHD. It can be used to help passengers on a flight as it reduces high altitude sickness. Ginkgo also improves alertness which is vital for exercises and sports. It boosts energy so it is recommended for athletes.

Furthermore, it helps with hair growth so it is advisable to use it alongside other hair products. Ginkgo helps with skin firming and smoothing. It works as an anti-aging and collagen producing agent. It retains moisture and reduces dryness in the skin. Ginkgo's anti-aging properties help retain a youthful and hydrated skin. It aids in weight loss because of the polyphenols and antioxidants properties. These properties improve insulin sensitivity which leads to weight loss. In addition to these, ginkgo has tyrosinase which develops pigmentation in the skin resulting in a lighter skin tone. Ginkgo also helps with eczema, acne, dermatitis and other skin related issues.

Antioxidants and anti-inflammatory properties found in ginkgo is the reason for its ability to reduce redness and puffiness in the skin. Ginkgo mixed together with pomegranate is a powerful combination because they slow down aging in human beings, stop brain dysfunction, increase blood flow to the system and kill some cancer cells. It is not advisable to take ginkgo with other medications like aspirin, warfarin etc. because taking ginkgo with these medications can interact with the medication.

Ginkgo boosts memory in people because it slows down or prevents age-related brain problems. It is a healthy plant-based supplement for albuminuria and other kidney functions which helps the kidney fight against diseases. Ginkgo is an effective treatment for anxiety, depression and extreme mood swings. It also fights off staphylococcus aureus and streptococcus pyogenes. Ginkgo has the capacity to treat hormonal imbalance therefore it is recommended for menopausal women as this can balance their estrogen levels and improve general menopausal symptoms.

5. Abronia Fragrans

This plant grows well in sandy soils, plains and pastures. It has hairy stems with flowers of green or pink color. Native Americans use this plant for their bowel problems and other diseases. In fact, they gave it a nickname "The Life medicine" because of its ability to increase appetite and lead to weight gain. Sometimes it was used as a cold lotion to treat mouth sores.

So abronia fragrans was used for years to kill certain ailments such as stomach ache, cold sores and also used to wash wounds as the anti-bacterial property in the plant ensured that wounds do not get infected. This plant was also used against insect bite and as an antidote for swallowing spiders. It was also used in aromatherapy for its sweet fragrance.

6. Acer Glabrum Var. Douglasii Aka Douglas Maple

The Douglas maple is a small tree found in some regions like Oregon State in America. It is also found in Alaska, Washington, Colorado, Arizona, and New Mexico. This plant is considered medicinal because of its chemical content. This plant was mostly used for curing diarrhea and as a general cure for several other diseases. The wood of the tree can be used to cure nausea and can also be used as a cathartic. It was also used to increase or promote the production of breast milk in nursing mothers. It was also taken by nursing mothers to heal the body post childbirth.

7. Box Elder

The box elder is a short-lived tree with compound leaves with about a 60-year lifespan.

The box elder plant was used by the Native Americans to induce vomiting, treat respiratory diseases, and also treat swellings, paralysis and other ailments.

It was also used for washing wounds in order to prevent them from getting infected. Due to its sugar content, it could be used as a substitute for other maple plants to make sugar. Box elder is edible and can be eaten boiled, roasted or even raw. The leaves can also be eaten raw or cooked. Box elder can be made into syrup or a drink. Box elder has also been used to make food for people and produce beverages and candies for children.

The leaves can be used to preserve other fruits or vegetables by wrapping the leaves around them. In addition to these medicinal benefits, the wood of box elder is also burnt as an incense to cleanse the environment of bad energy and allow positive thoughts to infiltrate the atmosphere in a room.

8. Silver Maple

The plant Acer Saccharinum is a plant native to so many regions in the United States. It is commonly called silver maple because of the silver underneath its leaves. Silver maple provides food and drinks for people because of its high sugar content. Silver maple is commonly used for making wooden objects like boxes, musical instruments and other small wooden objects. The Native Americans used silver maple to make cough medication. They also used it to treat cramps, dysentery and other diseases. They even used the water to wash sore eyes as it acted as a relief to the soreness. Silver maple also worked effectively as medication for menopausal women.

9. Black Cohosh

Black Cohosh is a plant native to North America and mainly found in the states of Ontario, Georgia and Kansas. Black Cohosh has certain medicinal properties that help in relieving menopausal symptoms in women. These properties include: nitrate, glycosides and triterpene. It is especially good for hot flashes and vaginal dryness, vertigo nervousness, irritation, heart palpitations and tinnitus. The herb is popularly known for reduction of hot flashes, restlessness and improvement in general quality of life.

Black Cohosh may take some weeks to have effects on menopausal symptoms but it is not advisable to take black cohosh for more than one year and prolonged use can cause some mild side effects like cramping, vaginal bleeding and weight gain. It is therefore advisable to speak with a doctor before using black cohosh as treatment for menopausal symptoms.

Although it may not directly increase sleep it will improve quality of sleep by dealing with the symptoms that give insomnia. These symptoms range from the hot flashes to all other menopausal symptoms that keep women awake at night. Black cohosh also reduces dryness in the vagina. It is also capable of reducing stress and anxiety.

Black Cohosh is beneficial for many health conditions but it is not advisable to take it together with aspirin, evening primrose oil, fish oil or alcohol. This is due to the fact that black cohosh interacts with them, which causes these medications not to have their full effect.

The reason why a person should not take black cohosh with alcohol is because alcohol contains ethanol which affects the liver. Black cohosh also affects the liver, so combining black cohosh with alcohol may be highly detrimental to the liver.

Black cohosh tries to balance the hormones that are being released during menopause. How does black cohosh work to balance the hormones during menopause? It works using its content called phytoestrogens. Phytoestrogens act like estrogen and increase the low estrogen level in menopausal women.

Though black cohosh reduces depression and anxiety especially during menopause, it is not advisable to take black cohosh if you have underlying health conditions like cancer, uterine fibroids, stroke, liver disease or when taking medications for high blood pressure. This is because black cohosh has a lot of effect on the hormones, so it could worsen these hormonal conditions. This herb can also induce ovulation in women because of the presence of phytoestrogens that affects the central nervous system.

In summary, black cohosh can regulate the menstrual cycle, tone the uterus and allow the shedding of the uterine lining. Black cohosh can also be used to treat kidney problems, depression, anxiety, nervousness, sore throat and other disorders such as abdominal problems etc.

10. Tall Hairy Agrimony

Agrimony is a medicinal herb that is used to heal various ailments. The seeds and the leaves are used to make medications.

This plant has a lot of medicinal benefits because of its high content of essential oil, vitamins and tannins which give the plants its medicinal value. This plant can be used to stop bleeding, cure gastric problems and treat diarrhea. It can also be used to heal skin problems, heal wounds and cuts by repairing the skin. In addition, the plant is good for curing uterine tract infection (UTI) and other urinary disorders. This herb can be taken in the form of tea or drink. To make this herbal tea, add the leaves and the stems to water to boil. Bring it to boil for five minutes. Then allow it to steep for ten minutes, stain and drink. You can also choose to apply it topically to the site.

This herb is also used for diarrhea, fever, liver infection, sore throat, irritable bowel syndrome, gallbladder disorder, cancer, tuberculosis, insomnia, excessive bleeding, stomach flu and diabetes. Agrimony plants are especially useful for children's ailments. It can be used to treat bladder leakage and to stop bedwetting.

Make tea out of this plant and sip the tea at least 30 minutes before going to bed. To make this tea, boil a cup of water and add a tablespoon of dried agrimony leaves and allow it to boil for 5 minutes. Turn off the heat and allow the leaves to steep in the hot water for 15 minutes, and drink about two cups per day. For sore throat, put the tea in your mouth and gargle for a few minutes.

This plant is helpful in reducing heavy menstruation. It also tones the membrane which alleviates coughs and sore throat. It can heal minor injuries when used to wash wounds and some skin conditions like eczema, dryness etc. It is really valuable to the digestive system as it aids digestion. Take this tea after a meal to aid digestion. It should be noted that this herb should not be used with some medication as it can interfere with the efficacy of those medications.

11. Ramp

Ramp is a species of onions that is native to North America. Ramp is also called Allium Tricoccum. This plant smells like garlic and a bit like onion. The plant can be used in place of onion in a recipe. Ramps are quite healthy because they are rich in vitamins, selenium and chromium because ramps have the capacity to improve eyesight, strengthen the bone and boost the immune and the cardiovascular system. The plant contains antioxidants which cleanse the body of toxins and free radicals that are harmful to the body.

However, due to its nutrient, ramp helps in weight loss, treats the digestive system, reduces inflammation, improves liver function, prevents heart disease and fights cancer. It prevents hypertension and normalizes the blood sugar levels in the body. Ramp also protects the brain and fights general infections due to its antibacterial property. As a result of its properties, ramp is considered a healthy meal. Its leaves are edible and medicinal. Ramp contains vitamin K which promotes blood clotting and better heart functions.

It reduces premenstrual syndrome, repairs tissues, absorbs iron and also increases collagen production which in turn helps the skin retain elasticity and youthful appearance. Ramps contain beta carotene which the body uses as vitamin A for better vision and cell communication. The antioxidants in ramps are essential for purging the body of harmful toxins that would have caused diseases in the body. This means that ramps prevent diseases from attacking the body. Ramp is a source of polyphenol antioxidants which protect the heart and also prevents some forms of cancer. It has sulphur compounds which reduces cholesterol and the formation of blood clots. It also helps in weight loss, digestion and general digestive system functions because of its fiber content. The allicin found in ramps has anti-cancer properties which mean that ramps also prevent cancer. The best part is that the ramp is readily available so a person can go ahead and add it to their meals to have a healthier diet.

12. White Alder

The white alder is a plant native to North America and used by the Native Americans for years to cure ailments. This plant is widely recognized for its medicinal benefits and nutritional content.

This plant's natural habitat is next to water bodies and is mostly found in Southern California, Colorado desert, Sierra, Nevada Montana, Washington and British Columbia. Native Americans mostly use this plant for problems pertaining to the female reproductive system which include menstruation, childbirth, lactation, menopause and every other medical condition peculiar to women.

The white alder was also used to treat stomach diseases, menstrual issues and for health care during childbirth. Furthermore, the white alder is used to treat inflammation of the throat and mouth. This is done by putting the white alder water in the mouth and gargling for a few minutes.

The plant's bark can be used to make balm for skin conditions like infected wounds, hemorrhoids, burns, eczema and ringworm. It has healing properties so once applied to the skin the white alder rids the body of blemishes and rejuvenates the skin. Its powder is used to treat skin infection, fever and other inflammation as it contains anti-inflammatory properties. It also prevents various kinds of cancer like breast and ovarian cancer.

13. Red Alder

The red alder belongs in the same family with the White album. The red alder is used to treat poison, insect bite and tuberculosis among other diseases. The red alder contains betulin and lupeol which fight against a number of tumors. As a result of its antitumor properties, the red alder prevents cancerous cells from growing.

The red alder can be differentiated from the white alder by the red color that forms on the bark when the tree is cut.

14. The California Sagebrush

The California sagebrush has been in existence in North America for hundreds of years. Like the white alder, this plant was used by the Native Americans to primarily treat women's health problems like menstrual cramps, heavy bleeding, gestational diseases and menopausal symptoms. The women take the herb regularly just before their menstruation. They also used it to induce labor. This plant was also used to quicken labor.

The Native Americans used this plant to prevent cold, cough, sore throat, fever and can be used as pain reliever for sores in the mouth. In addition, it was used to treat rheumatism, arthritis and for relief for asthma by adding it in the bath water for topical use and ingested for internal use.

The sagebrush can also be used for aromatherapy as it contains terpene chemicals which give it a sweet fragrance. The plant can also be used to treat insect bite as it acts as a relief to the sting. The leaves of this plant are anti-microbial so when the leaves are burned and inhaled, it clears the upper respiratory system of diseases like bronchitis, sore throat, sinus infections and other infections.

The flavonoids in the plants are anti-inflammatory because they penetrate the skin and relieve inflammation. It stimulates the muscles in the uterine tract and it was believed to hasten and reduce labor pains. The two chemicals contained in sagebrush are monoterpenoids and flavonoids. The flavonoids are anti-inflammatory and the monoterpenoids are the reason for the plant's sweet aroma and pain-relieving effect.

15. California Mugwort

The California Mugwort was used by Native Americans to relieve pains in the joints, rheumatism, headache, chest pain, bruises and rashes. It was also used as an abortifacient to either abort or prevent pregnancies. Native Americans also used this plant as treatment for bronchitis, arthritis, insect repellent and negative energy repellent.

California Mugwort is also called the dream plant as it treats mild insomnia. This is achieved by drinking the tea made from this plant or by putting some of its leaves in diffusers and inhaling it to get better rest. This plant is also used to promote blood circulation so it promotes a calm and wholesome state of mind and body. The tea is used to treat hysteria, epilepsy, irregular periods and convulsion in children. It is also used to stimulate the gastric juices in the tummy for proper digestion, so this plant is useful to the digestive system.

To make the tea, put 3 teaspoons of leaves into one cup of boiling water and let it boil for 10 minutes. Then allow it to steep in the water for an extra 10 minutes in order to get all of the nutrients out of the leaves. After it has steeped for 10 minutes, strain the leaves out and drink the tea. Mugwort is an anti-inflammatory, anti-tumor, antifungal, anticoagulant and antidiabetic herb.

However, it is advisable not to take mugwort with blood-thinning medications as it could make the blood really thin. As an anti-tumor, mugwort plant fights against cancer and because of its antioxidant properties it prevents free radicals from harming the skin. The extract of this plant can be used to make cream to cleanse the eyes, hydrate the skin and nourish the hair. This plant promotes a glowing complexion and a hydrated skin.

16. White Sagebrush

The White sagebrush is a plant native to North America. The Native Americans use this plant because of its medicinal benefit and serves as protections against negative energies. It is also applied topically for skin conditions and also as medicine for cold, fever, cough and other diseases of the upper respiratory system. In addition, it treats excessive sweating and indigestion. If a person experiences frequent sinus infections, such a person can drink white sage regularly to stop the infections for good. The white sage has eucalyptol which kills bacteria and has the minty effect that clears and soothes the sinus.

White sage tea relieves indigestion and diarrhea. It also reduces mucus in the throat and the lungs which leads to a reduction in the common cold. The white sage drink also relieves menstruation cramps. It also lowers cholesterol levels and has an anti-obesity effect which means that hypertension and other heart problems get reduced through the use of white sage.

The white sage is also used to make incense because of its fragrance. It is burned for religious rituals or personal aromatherapy for a cleaner atmosphere.

17. Giant Cane

The giant cane is native to the South Central and Southeastern United States. The Giant cane was used by Native Americans to cure diseases in the liver, the digestive system and in the upper respiratory system. The tea made out of this plant has tonic properties for the gastrointestinal system. Also, this plant has been used to treat bloating ulcer gastritis and so many other things.

However, to treat headache, make a paste of the root of this plant and apply topically to the forehead. The paste relaxes the muscles and relieves the headache.

18. Canada Wild Ginger

This plant is used to create a strong flavor in food and seasoning and also act as medication for different ailments. The Native Americans use these plants to cure various ailments like digestive system problems, upper respiratory system problems, fever, cramps and other menstrual issues. It also cures headaches, convulsions, asthma, tuberculosis, urinary tract infections, urinary disorders, swollen breasts and sexually transmitted diseases. The plant is mainly used to treat intestinal ailment, relieve stomach aches, menstrual cramps as well as indigestion. It is also used to treat colic and that is why it is also popularly referred to as the colic root.

19. Whorled Milkweed

This plant is used by Native Americans to cure snake bite and respiratory tract problems. True to its name, it is used to promote milk production in nursing mothers. Milkweed is considered a medicinal plant because it treats diseases in the lungs.

Milkweed is a natural painkiller and acts as a form of treatment for diarrhea. Also, the milkweed was used to treat rheumatism and pleurisy. The plant was also given to women after childbirth to help their reproductive system to go back to normal. A person can make use of the milk for treatment of asthma, fever, rashes and swelling. It is worthy to note that the plant is potentially poisonous, so one has to be careful with planting milkweed or keeping it around the house where children or pets can get to it.

20. Desert Broom

It is a plant native to North America and it is found in California, Arizona, New Mexico and Texas. Native Americans use this plant to make a drink which was used to treat headaches, general body pains, joint pains, rheumatism, sore muscles, arthritis, colic and sinus infections. This plant contains flavonoids called luteolin which has anti-inflammatory, antifungal and antioxidant properties. The herb is capable of reducing cholesterol levels in the body. Desert broom should be applied topically for sore muscles, that is, it should be used to massage the muscles. Exercise caution when taking this herbal tea because some parts of the desert broom are poisonous to humans.

21. Arrowleaf Balsamroot

Arrowleaf balsamroot is a beautiful plant native to North America of the sunflower tribe. This plant is well known in the United States and Canada for its beauty and its medicinal uses. In traditional medicine the arrowleaf balsamroot helps in pain reliefs in wound dressing and healing of bruises. The root is often taken as tea to treat cough, cold, fever, tuberculosis and other illnesses. Arrowleaf can also be inhaled through a diffuser.

22. Evening Primrose

The evening primrose is a yellow flower that grows in North America and part of Europe. This flower is known for balancing hormonal issues and also for wound healing.

The evening primrose is a plant common in Florida, Alberta and Texas. This plant is widely recognized for its medicinal and dietary benefits. This plant is capable of curing menopause symptoms, arthritis, skin conditions and so many other conditions. It can be taken orally or applied topically. However, for eczema and other skin conditions, primrose should be put topically on the skin. Also, when it is used for hair growth primrose should be applied and massaged into the scalp. The famous primrose oil helps to regulate blood flow and to treat menopausal symptoms. Taking primrose oil for a week greatly reduces anxiety and other social disorders. Evening primrose is also used for treating wounds and other skin bruises. Primrose greatly reduces menopausal symptoms like hot flashes, night sweats, difficulty in sleeping, vaginal dryness and mood swings. Evening primrose also reduces breast pain; this is achieved by reducing the inflammation and preventing prostaglandins that cause breast pain. Evening primrose also moisturizes the skin and keeps it hydrated. Apply evening primrose topically to keep your skin looking well nourished, moisturized and cared for.

For gestation and in preparation for labor, evening primrose oil is usually sold in capsules so when asked to use for these issues, you could either be advised to swallow or insert the oil into the vagina to soften and prepare the cervix for labor. As an anti-inflammatory herb you could drink the oil directly to help cure inflammation in the body. Evening primrose is just like fish and flax oil when it comes to Omega 6 fatty acids, this means that evening primrose can help cure infertility issues.

Evening primrose is also good for certain health conditions like asthma, hepatitis b, high cholesterol, psoriasis, psoriatic arthritis, breast pain, liver cancer and many others. Evening primrose can also manage or prevent the following diseases: chronic fatigue, diaper rash, infant development, pregnancy complications, rheumatism, arthritis, schizophrenia, cancer, cold, acne, heart disease, Alzheimer's disease and ulcerative colitis.

It should be noted that evening primrose may interact with medication so a person taking blood thinning medication for instance, do not mix it with evening primrose oil as it may cause bleeding because evening primrose is an anticoagulant. Also, people with some nerve issues like epilepsy and other seizures should not take evening primrose to avoid having seizures or other side effects. Before taking evening primrose, speak to a doctor.

23. Devil's Club

The devil's club is a North American plant of the ginseng family with large leaves and sharp prickles. This club is mainly planted for its medicinal benefits

The devil's club is used in America as a medicinal plant. The root and the stem are what are mostly used for medicine. The fruits of the devil's club are not edible for human consumption. The devil's club produces a balm which is used to treat arthritis, rheumatism, fever, tuberculosis, stomach ache, cancer, cough, sore throat, diabetes, low blood sugar and pneumonia. It can also be used as a purging medicine. It should be noted that the devil's club plant is partly edible while some parts are poisonous to humans, so care should be exercised during consumption.

The devil's club helps in treating eczema and other skin related issues. This is due to the fact that the devil's club has antioxidant and anti-inflammatory properties which help it to heal surface wounds and other skin defects. It is worthy of note that the devil's club leaves have more anti-tumor, flavonoids and phenolic content than the root and stem. This means that the leaves have higher antioxidant content and the antioxidant is used for preventing harmful radicals from harming the human body.

Native Americans used the devil's club to stop the flow of breast milk during weaning. They also used it to fight upper respiratory diseases and digestion problems. The devil's club is also drunk after childbirth to restore a woman's body back to its normal state. The devil's club has a compound called sesquiterpenes which is anti-rheumatism, anti-cholesterol and anti-inflammatory. This means that the devil's claw can effectively reduce inflammation, rheumatism and cholesterol levels in the body. They also balance the body stress levels. Oil made from this herb is effective in fighting against psoriasis.

24. Echinacea

The Echinacea plant is a genus in the daisy family. This plant has like 10 different species and is mostly found in Eastern and central North America. This plant has been used for hundreds of years by the Native Americans to heal ailment and prevent some diseases. People often use the plant to shorten the period of time for cold and flu and other upper respiratory tract diseases. The plant is great for fighting infections and boosting the immune system because of its high vitamin content. In addition, it has a large amount of antioxidant, anti-inflammatory and anti-viral properties. It is best known for its effect on the immune system. Like we said earlier the plant is perfect for boosting the immune system by increasing the white blood cells which helps to fight numerous infections and viruses. This plant therefore makes a person recover faster from any illness.

In addition, it reduces the symptoms of cold and the severity of upper respiratory tract problems. The plant can be taken as tea twice daily for the first few days after infection has taken place. It could also be used as prevention against infections. Many people confirmed that this plant is as effective as over-the-counter medication when it comes to fighting flu, the common cold, fever and such other diseases. A person can even take this plant together with vitamin C as there is no interaction between the two.

The herb is also best for preventive measures so if a person suspects a cold is coming up, such a person can simply drink this tea a few days before the cold and it will be effectively treated. This plant is majorly used against bacterial and viral infections. It can also act as a pain reliever because of its anti-inflammatory properties. It can lower pain and help in treating sinus infections.

It is an antioxidant so it moisturizes the skin, gets rid of free radicals that could be harmful to the skin and protects the skin from the sun rays. It also keeps the protective layer of the skin strong so that moisture is locked inside the body. This herb contains properties that help create white blood cells which are needed to fight infections. It is not advisable to take this herb on an empty stomach because of its powerful nature. Instead, a person should take it immediately after eating or at least with a full glass of water. The extract of this plant boosts the immune system which makes the body stand up against germs.

It also works for antiviral respiratory problems. It does not only help with flu, it also treats the symptoms of flu. The Native Americans use this herb not just for respiratory problems but to treat infections and wounds. This herb is also good for the stomach as it helps balance the good bacteria in the stomach. This plant moisturizes skin by increasing the levels of lipids in the body like ceramides and epidermal lipids which keep the body strong and prevent escape of moisture. It is antioxidant so it helps defend the body against toxics which result in a healthier body.

It should be noted that although this herb is perfect for flu and cold a person should avoid it if such a person is dealing with high blood pressure as there is risk of it increasing high blood pressure.

25. Goldenseal

Goldenseal is a thick yellow knitted rootstock plant native to North America. This plant is used for a lot of medicinal benefits. It is used for treatment of the common cold and other upper respiratory tract issues like sinus infections, cold, and fever. It also treats the digestive system like stomach ache, swelling, peptic ulcer, diarrhea, intestinal gas, hemorrhoids, constipation etc.

Goldenseal really works because of its antibacterial properties which reduces bad bacteria in the body. Goldenseal also cures sinus infections, menstrual cramps, heavy menstruation, skin disorders and other inflammatory diseases. It treats skin infections, removes blemishes and tones the skin pigmentation.

This herb has basically the same types of chemical compounds that turmeric has, so goldenseal is also anti-inflammatory, antibacterial and antioxidant. This means that just like turmeric, goldenseal is good for skin problems, wound healing, inflammatory issues, and other sinus infections in the body.

Goldenseal also has immune-boosting properties, so this plant can boost the immune system to fight against diseases. Goldenseal being a natural antibacterial and antibiotics can be used for oral care. It can be used as a mouthwash to keep the teeth, mouth and gums in good condition. Some people also say that goldenseal can be used for uterine tract infection but there is not much evidence to support this. Goldenseal can be applied topically on the skin to cure rashes, eczema, dryness, sores and bruises in the mouth. It can also be applied around the gums in the mouth for some minutes then rinsed out to help heal gum infections. However, there are some points to be noted, pregnant women and nursing mothers should stay away from goldenseal as goldenseal can have some negative side effects on the baby.

26. Grape Seed Extract

Grape seed is a medicinal herb used for curing a lot of ailments. Grape seed oil is used for weight loss. Being rich in vitamin E, grapeseed is an antioxidant that helps repair the skin, flush out toxins that can destroy the body, rejuvenate the skin, fight cancer, help with varicose veins and grow the hair. It helps to remove free radicals from the body and prevent the growth of harmful bacteria in the body. Grape seed oil is good for the skin and the scalp as it heals dryness, unclog pores and removes dead cells which allows for hair growth and healthier skin. Apply grape seed oil on the face at night and let it stay overnight to rejuvenate the skin. As a result of the presence of polyphenols in grape seed oil, the oil is able to slow down the aging process and also reverse the symptoms of aging on the human skin. These include wrinkles, saggy skin and stretch marks. It gives skin an elasticity and plumpness that helps retain a youthful look.

The use of grape seed oil for 2 weeks can make great changes to the face. Grape seed oil can also be used for wounds because the oil has anti-inflammatory properties which heals wounds and reduces scarring as much as possible. Grape seed oil does not only tone the skin, it also tightens it to make it look healthier and firmer. Also, grape seed oil on the lips can eradicate dryness, weakness and lip lines. Grape seed oil can also be used as a cleanser for the face. Massage this oil into your face for about five minutes in a circular massage until your face feels warm. Allow it to sit for about 10 minutes then wash it off. People that are prone to acne have linoleic deficiency. Grape seed oil has high content of linoleic acid this means that grape seed oil when applied regularly to this acne-prone face will prevent acne because of the infiltration of linoleic acid in the face.

Grape seed extract reduces risk of cancer and cardiovascular diseases. It also inhibits the storage of fat, it also gives energy, and surges metabolism to burn fat. Grape seed extract also prevents cavities in the mouth, prevents cancer, cardiovascular diseases, varicose veins and retina diseases.

27. Cranberry

Cranberry is a fruit that has been used for hundreds of years to cure different ailments. Cranberries have medicinal benefits which prevent, manage and cure diseases. This is due to the fact that cranberries are high in antioxidant content. It also has anti-inflammatory and anti-fungal anti-viral content. So, what's the benefit of cranberry? It slows down the aging process, keeps the heart in good condition, prevents urinary tract infection, boosts immunity by improving the white blood cells and reduces menopausal symptoms. Cranberry also prevents some kinds of cancer and lowers blood pressure in people with hypertension. Cranberry is helpful for the kidney and also helps the urinary tract. This is because the fruit has certain properties called proanthocyanidins. This property prevents bacteria from growing in the urinary tract therefore preventing bacteria from causing diseases in the urinary tract. Cranberry also helps in boosting collagen production due to its high content of vitamin C. This helps to moisturize the body and improve the elasticity of the skin, making it ready to bounce back after pregnancy and other changes. This elasticity slows down the aging process.

Cranberries are also good for the brain because of their nutrients called polyphenols. Polyphenols are good for brain function and also protects the brain from diseases. Due to its anti-inflammatory properties, cranberry is good for the scalp and hair. The fruit removes blemishes, scars and rash and allows for a healthier scalp and better hair growth. Cranberry flushes the kidney by cleaning the lining of any bacteria that would have caused infections in the kidney. Cranberry, being rich in vitamin C helps in fortifying the immune system. It also fights free radicals and other harmful toxins from residing in the body. Cranberries help with dehydration and constipation, so drinking a glass of cranberry can help the easy passage of feces through the body.

28. Umbellata

Umbellata plant is a small tree that is native to rainforest. This plant is highly medicinal as it helps to treat various ailments that afflict the human body such as blood deficiency, swelling, diabetes mellitus, obesity and infections. Umbellata plant has anti-inflammatory and anti-bacterial properties which help fight infections. The plant is also used to treat liver problems, worms, fever, leprosy, sores and several other diseases. Umbellata also helps with male infertility as it is said to successfully combat infertility in men.

29. Mayflower

The Mayflower plant has a lot of medicinal benefits especially to Native Americans. It was used as an antiseptic and also used for bladder stones, prostatitis, cystitis and other urinary tract infections. The leaves of this flower act as a diuretic and so it helps the body to get rid of water and salt. This decreases the amount of liquids that go through the body thereby reducing blood pressure. The removal of extra fluids can also result in weight loss. If a person is battling with dehydration, the person should avoid mayflower tea.

30. Tea Tree

Tea tree oil is one of the most important essential oils in the world of natural remedies. This oil is famous for its antibacterial, anti-viral, anti-fungal and anti-inflammatory contents.

This oil is used to treat skin diseases like acne and eczema, scalp problems like dryness, dandruff and lice infestation. Due to its antibacterial properties, tea-tree oil can also be used as hand sanitizer, as an insect repellent, for wound healing and to get rid of nail fungus. This oil can also be used as deodorant and as a mouthwash.

The tea tree oil can be applied topically as it seldom causes irritation for the skin so it doesn't need carrier oil. This oil can be applied regularly on the skin with little to no side effects for most people. If a person notices any bad reaction to tea tree oil, such a person should stop applying it until he/she speaks with a physician. Tea tree oil also lightens the skin because it kills acne so it penetrates the skin and prevents clogging.

As a result of its antiseptic content, tea tree oil cures itchy scalp and skin and also soothes irritations and wounds on the skin.

Tea trees are also good for eye treatment. These antibacterial antifungal properties treat the eye and other infections. Place a bag on the eye for 30 minutes until you notice a relief in your symptoms. Also, you can apply tea tree oil on the eyelashes for the same effect. Tea tree oil is anti-aging because it balances the oil content in the body, shrinks pores, repairs and moisturizes skin. This oil also tightens the skin and makes it firmer which is best for saggy or aging skin. In addition, tree oil also smoothens the skin and prevents wrinkles. Lastly, it also deals with insect bite by reducing the inflammation and infection.

31. Flax Seed

Flax seeds are highly nutritious seeds with so many medicinal benefits. Flax seeds are rich in Omega-3 fat, dietary fiber, protein and lignans which fight against cancer. Therefore, flax seeds lower cholesterol levels, reduces high blood pressure and prevents some heart diseases.

Flaxseed is healthy for the digestive system as it helps with constipation and improves general digestive health. Due to the fibrous content, flaxseed helps with constipation and the easy passage of fecal matter through the colon. Flaxseed also helps with fat as it can lead to weight loss or reduction. Flaxseed can be used for belly fat reduction, simply mix grounded flaxseed in hot water, boil for 5 minutes and drink. This helps in weight loss and also to build immunity in the body as flaxseed is a good source of vitamin.

As a result of the high content of Vitamin D and B which helps in hair growth, it can make a person's hair grow longer and faster. Flaxseed being rich in protein and fiber helps in weight loss. As fiber helps someone feel full for longer and acts as a suppressant for appetite. Flaxseed is also low in carbohydrates and sugar which means that they are low in calories. Flaxseed is especially good for women because it is rich in Omega-3 fatty acids.

A person can take flaxseed as tea or add its oil as salad dressing. Flaxseed can also be made into pastries or just drink them in water. For weight loss purposes, flaxseed should be eaten before meals as this creates a feeling of fullness which makes people feel less hungry for food. This will lead to a reduction in food intake and finally lead to weight loss.

Flaxseeds are high in antioxidants because it rids the body of free radicals, prevents blemishes and signs of aging on the face by keeping the skin moisturized and smoothen out. It prevents sagging as it tightens the skin. It also prevents diarrhea. It helps to keep a glowing skin. Flaxseed is especially good for women because of its phytoestrogen content that resembles the estrogen content in women. This means that flaxseeds can regularize periods and hormonal imbalances. Flaxseed gel can be used to tighten skin, plump the lips and give it a more youthful appearance. Flax seeds increase women's fertility rate, normalize hormones and reduce the risk of cancer in women. Flaxseed also reduces some symptoms of menopause in women like hot flashes and restlessness. Flaxseed regulates estrogen production in the body by supplying lignin to the body. Lignin is known to promote estrogen production which regularizes menstruation and promotes fertility in women. Flaxseed also helps in maintaining a healthy ovary. To achieve this, take a tablespoon of flaxseed for 3 days then increase to 2 tablespoons for the next three days. On the 7th day, increase to 3 tbsp and take this regularly for 11 weeks and the progress should be noted in a journal.

32. Chia Seed

Chia seed is known for its low calories and high nutritional value. This seed helps with weight loss, constipation and digestion. Chia seeds regularize the bowel movement by reducing constipation and helping fight against colon infections. Chia seeds are one of the best nuts known for weight loss because of its omega-3 content, it is good for boosting the digestive system metabolism and generally uses up energy in order to help one lose fat.

To get the most out of chia seeds, consume chia seeds water in the morning to regulate the digestive system and help with bowel movement. Because chia seed is high in fiber, it makes you feel full even before taking the first meal in the day. This means that you're going to eat smaller portions and stay satisfied for longer periods because of the fibrous contents of chia. Chia seed can be added to meals, smoothies and drinks to provide a healthier diet. One way to consume chia seeds for weight loss is by substituting chia seeds flour for normal flour.

As a result of the omega-3 content, chia seeds help set up a barrier that retains the skin moisture and keeps the skin youthful and nourished. It contains antioxidants which flush out harmful toxins and fight free radicals in the body. Chia seeds absorb water which softens stool and makes for easier passage.

33. Erigenia Bulbosa.

It is a hermaphrodite plant native to North America. This plant which belongs to the carrot family has been declared endangered species. Due to its anti-inflammatory properties, the Native Americans usually chewed this plant as a panacea for their tooth ache.

34. Yerba Santa

The yerba Santa plant was regarded as a sacred plant by the Native Americans mainly because of its medicinal powers and ability to clear the atmosphere of bad energy and release positive energies in its place.

The yerba Santa plant is mainly used for respiratory problems. This plant is used to clear mucus in the nose. It is also taken for headaches, migraines, muscle pains, arthritis, chronic bronchitis, cough, cold, tuberculosis, asthma, fever and dry mouth.

Apart from the fuses the plant was also used to cure digestive system problems, skin problems and sexually transmitted diseases. So, this plant was regarded as a panacea for almost every kind of disease. This was because of the anti-bacterial, anti-inflammatory and antioxidant properties present in the plant. Today the plants can still be used for respiratory related diseases.

Simply put the leaves of this plant into boiling water and allow it to boil for 10 minutes. Turn off the heat and let the leaves steep in the water for about 10 minutes. After 10 minutes strain the leaves out and drink the water. It should be noted that it is best to take this plant when it is relatively young because its nutritional value is at its peak in the young green shoots and other parts of the young plant. When it is old and dry, the plant loses some of its active properties.

35. White Gourd

The white gourd plant is good for GERD. White gourd plant also helps with acid reflux and heartburn. The plant contains vitamins, protein and sucrose. It has cooling properties so it helps reduce heat in the body. With its alkaline nature it also acts as a natural coolant for the body. It lowers heart rate, aids in weight loss, detoxifies the kidney and helps prevent some heart diseases.

To detoxify the kidney, take it early in the morning before breakfast. This will make it flush germs and toxins out of the body. It is also a good source of carotene and flavonoids which are antioxidants that prevent the growth of free radicals and other toxins that are harmful to the body. It helps the body maintain a youthful glow. This plant prevents diabetes and heart diseases. You can take white gourd as a drink to see all these positive changes.

36. Calypso

Calypso is a plant native to North America. Calypso is sometimes called helium beans. These plants are edible and low in calories and fat. Calypso's medicinal benefits include lowering cholesterol. Due to its high antioxidant content it boosts the immune system and prevents some diseases especially upper respiratory tract diseases like cold, flu, fever, headache, sore throat and minor sinus infections. Calypso has fiber so it fills people up for longer, curbs food cravings, suppresses appetite which leads to weight loss.

The fiber also helps the colon as it prevents bacteria from growing in the colon when allowing the good bacteria take over. It also reduces the risk of rectal cancer. Calypso has enzymes that fight against cancer. Therefore eating calypso beans lowers your risk of having certain types of cancer. Calypso also stabilizes blood sugar; it helps maintain a balance in the blood sugar levels of the body. Calypso also helps with heart diseases because of its potassium and magnesium content which relaxes blood vessels and allows blood flow better. It also has anti-inflammatory properties which reduces inflammation of the heart and prevents heart attack. Calypso also helps in constipation due to its high fiber content. It allows food to move freely along the intestine to the colon which aids digestion. Calypso boosts the immune system because of its high amount of zinc magnesium copper iron. This means that it prevents anemia and other diseases of the blood. So, calypso is an all-round good plant that promotes good health, prevents diseases and sometimes cures diseases in the body.

37. Almond

Almonds with its high protein, fiber, fat, vitamin and magnesium contents are one of the best nuts for lowering cholesterol, diabetes, obesity and high blood pressure.

Almonds contain vitamin E and antioxidants because almonds are high in antioxidants and vitamin E. It is one of the best oils for the skin. It also helps in weight loss because almonds have a high fiber content which makes a person feel full for a longer period of time.

To use almonds for weight loss, eat the nuts like 20 minutes before your meal. You can also take it in a drink or add it to your pastries. Almonds can also be eaten raw as it regulates blood sugar and boosts metabolism. Almond flour can be used as a substitute for baking. This will greatly reduce diabetes, mellitus, high blood pressure and other diseases.

38. Basil

Basil is an herb used for cooking and medicine. This herb is native to Asia but used all over the world for medicinal purposes. Basil is used to cure stomach ache, kidney problems, gas, worms, infections, common cold, upper respiratory problems, loss of appetite, snake venom and insect bite. Basil has properties like eugenol, lineonol and citronellol which fight infections and inflammations. These compounds are anti-inflammatory in nature so they are used to fight inflammation like heart disease and digestive tract issue arthritis. As a result of the presence of antibacterial properties, it is used to fight bacteria in the body. Basil also contains vitamin K, vitamin A and vitamin C. It has Omega-3 fatty acids, magnesium, calcium, iron and magnesium. Basil can be used to treat injuries and skin infections and generally keep the wounds from getting infected. Basil can be added to food, taken as a drink, inhaled or steamed through diffusers or hot water. It is also used to treat kidney stones because the compounds normalize uric acid levels in the body which prevents kidney stones. Basil is also good for metabolic stress as it can help with weight loss and lowering of cholesterol levels.

Basil treats upper respiratory problems, sinus infections, loosening mucus and clearing the windpipe. To use basil for this purpose, add some leaves to boiling water or add the essential oil to boiling water. Let it boil for 5 minutes, turn off the heat and allow it to steep for 10 minutes. Pour into a bowl, place the bowl under your face, cover your head with clothes and inhale the steam for about 10 minutes to loosen mucus and stop cold.

Basil oil can be added to diffusers for fresher air. The oil can be used to cure anxiety, depression and fatigue. If you are feeling down, add the oil to diffusers in the room and inhale it for about an hour. Basil has the capacity to lighten someone's mood and calm the nerves. If there is no diffuser, spray basil oil on a clean handkerchief and put it close to your nose.

Basil oil can also be used to treat acne, cough, gout and bronchitis. Basil is especially good for the skin as it is high in vitamin A, C, K, copper and fat. Mix basil oil with a carrier oil like coconut or jojoba oil. Rub basil oil on the face and let it stay for 5 minutes. Wash it off and wipe the face clean with a face towel. Basil boosts the metabolism in the body which aids in weight loss, so it helps burn calories faster and converts food into energy. To use Basil for weight loss, wash basil leaves and boil, allow it to boil for 5 minutes. Let it stay in the water for an extra 10 minutes in order to get the full nutrients in the water. Pour into a cup, add a slice of lemon and drink.

39. Bay Leaves

Bay leaves are aromatic herbs that are mostly used for cooking and add flavor to food. Most people just use bay leaves for food and stew because of its nice aroma but there is more to this herb than the flavor it adds to food. Bay leaves are actually medicinal to the body being that it is rich in vitamin A and C, potassium, calcium, magnesium and iron.

People who cook with bay leaves may not know this but it promotes good health. Here are some medicinal benefits of this wonderful herb that has graced our kitchens for hundreds of years. Bay leaves help with migraine as it reduces migraine effectively. Also, bay leaves reduce cholesterol. With its ability to reduce urea in the body, bay leaves can prevent the formation of kidney stones in the kidney. It can heal wounds because of its antioxidant, antibacterial and antiviral properties. Bay leaves even act as an insect repellent and an anticonvulsant medication. Bay leaves help with digestion problems. Bay leaves also improve insulin and glucose metabolism because of the presence of polyphenol which controls glucose levels in the body. Their leaves being loaded with antioxidants, helps with hair growth. Some people even use bay leaves to make their hair wash. To use it, boil bay leaves for 20 minutes and use it to wash the hair for a better shine.

40. Rosemary

One of the most popular herbs in America is the Rosemary and it is also called salvia rosmarinus. The rosemary has been used as a spice for so many years, it has been added to stews, soups and salad to improve their flavor. But apart from this, the rosemary is also medicinal as it helps with a lot of health conditions. Rosemary is popularly known for improving memory, aids digestion, reduces hair loss, helps with inflammation like arthritis, rheumatism and several other conditions. As a result of its anti-inflammatory and antioxidant compounds, the rosemary is perfect for immune system boost and better blood circulation. It is also known to heighten alertness and focus in people. People take Rosemary tea to boost their immune system and reduce harmful bacteria in the digestive tract. Rosemary contains carnosic acid which improves good bacteria in the body and reduces harmful bacteria, toxins and free radicals in the body.

To make the rosemary tea, put 10 leaves of Rosemary in boiling water and let it boil for 5 minutes. Turn off the heat and let it steep in the water for 10 minutes. Pour it into a cup then add a slice of lemon or tablespoon of honey and drink.

41. Chamomile

Chamomile is a plant in the daisy family that is usually used in America for traditional medicine. Most people take chamomile tea for anxiety, depression, pain relief, inflammation, blood sugar levels, cancer treatment, cold, other respiratory problems, sleep and relaxation. Chamomile is largely recognized as a mild sedative. Its properties help induce sleep and give a calm feeling. The calming effect of chamomile comes from a certain property in the plant called apigenin. This property decreases anxiety and induces sleep. Chamomile is also good for constipation as it relaxes the intestinal muscles allowing it to pass poo. It is a stress reliever so take this tea whenever you feel really stressed.

Chamomile is not only good for stress; it also helps with weight loss because of its appetite reducing properties. It especially relaxes the muscles and flushes out toxins from the body. It also prevents diabetes and other kidney diseases. Its sesquiterpene lactones content gives a liver detoxification. Chamomile can be taken in the form of tea or inhaled from a diffuser by simply adding drops of chamomile oil in the diffuser and inhaling for a good night's rest.

Chamomile is also good for hormonal disorders as it helps balance the hormones and regularize periods in women. It has properties that help trigger estrogen production in the body, so this can normalize hormones and regulate periods which help women with fertility problems.

Apart from this, chamomile is also good for the skin because of its healing properties. It is capable of healing wounds, ulcers and sores. It also reduces irritation in eczema and rashes. It can also treat dandruff and dryness in the scalp.

42. Virginia Spring Beauty

The Virginia spring beauty is a flower that is native to North America. It can be used to treat convulsions and act as a contraceptive. It has also been used to treat eyesight problems, sore throat, skin dryness, dandruff, urinary tract problems and digestive problems. This plant being rich in vitamin A and C boosts the immune system and prevents diseases.

43. Ephedra Californica.

Ephedra Californica is a medicinal herb that contains different healing properties like alkaloids, ephedrine and other stimulants. These properties stimulate the brain, increase metabolism and heightens heart rate. It also acts as an antidepressant and an anti-decongestant as it lowers depression and anxiety in people. It also keeps people alert. This plant gives a surge of energy therefore acting as an energy booster for people. It should be noted that people with some underlying heart condition should not use this herb as it could have adverse effects on their health.

44. Erythrina Herbacea.

Erythrina Herbacea is a plant majorly found in South Louisiana and in other states in the United States. Although part of this plant is medicinal and edible, others are toxic and hallucinogenic. The flowers and young leaves are considered edible and medicinal, so it can be used to cure or manage several elements but some other part of the plant is considered poisonous and can lead to some bad health conditions or even death. The seed of the plant can be used topically for rheumatic pain. The root was used by Native Americans for digestive problems and stomach ache.

45. Bigleaf Aster.

Bigleaf aster was used by the Native Americans as blood tonic. The leaves and roots of the plants were used for medicine for headache, stomach ache, joint ache, laxative and sexually transmitted diseases.

CHAPTER TWO: HOW TO INCORPORATE NATIVE AMERICAN MEDICINE IN OUR MODERN LIVES

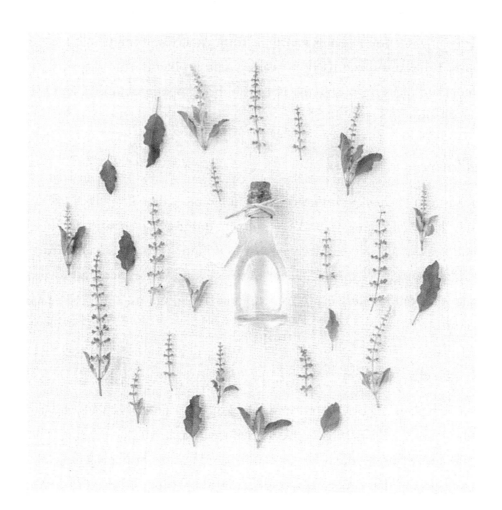

For hundreds of years, human beings have used plants as medication to cure their different ailments. Some of these plants were also used in cooking, and others were not. The early Americans were of Indian descent, and most of their traditional medicine emanated from ancient practices. Due to the lack of science and technology, these people had to rely on animal behavior trial and error to get answers to their ailment. In today's world, science and technology seem to have taken over in the treatment of various ailments.

The advantage science has is that it gives precise dosage, considers individual health conditions and unique diagnoses of each person, while traditional medicine seems to be in general and not really tested to know how it works for each individual needs. In the olden days, it was better because the medicine man lived in the community, so he knew all the members of the community he served. This helped him to diagnose each person based on his knowledge of the person and the history of the person's ailment. Now the medicine man seems to be an archaic practice as more people turn to science for solutions to their different ailments.

Another reason more people seem to favor science is that science and technology seem quicker and produce more results than traditional medicine in this fast world. Traditional medicine often requires patience and consistency to work. On the other hand, science seems to give faster results in a shorter time. Even with all these, a lot of people still want to go back to the traditional ways of treating diseases and would like to know how to incorporate this Native American medicine into their modern everyday lives. First, always speak to a doctor about any traditional supplements you are taking to do his research and tell you if there will be any problems or interactions between any medication you might be on and the herbal supplements you want to start.

Another way to incorporate traditional medicine is by adding it to your diet. Most of these herbs are for the prevention of diseases, so they have to be taken regularly even when there is nothing obviously wrong with the person. They also have to be taken in the right dosage and over a period of time to see resolved results. Before a person embarks on adding any herb to their diet, do adequate research on it and know possible side effects. This is because some herbs, no matter how good they are, come with some side effects if taken beyond a period of time.

The good part of traditional medicine is that it tries to give wholeness, not just a cure to a certain disease. People still continue to use traditional medicine side-by-side with modern medicine because they can easily coexist to give better results than just relying on modern medicine. Modern medicine simply tests traditional medicine and tries to make them more effective, work within a shorter time frame, and regularize the dosage. So traditional medicine is basically what modern medicine is made of. But in this situation, it is produced in laboratories, and some chemicals and preservatives are added to make them more effective and last longer.

 Some pharmaceuticals may try to downgrade the effect or the effectiveness of traditional medicine. However, it has been seen and proven that traditional medicine is very effective in treating physical, psychological diseases. In America, lots of people turn to modern medicine in other parts of the world. Like in a lot of African countries, people still rely on traditional medicine for major ailments. This is because traditional medicine is cheaper, has little or no side effects, and is fresher.

So traditional medicine works well and can be incorporated in today's world to give a person not just a cure but wholeness. Like I said before, traditional medicines are both curative and preventive. So, to achieve wholeness, traditional medicine is best incorporated in diet and beauty regimens. This is because of modern medicine in the sense that you cannot take aspirin, for instance, daily, to prevent headaches without abusing the medication. But in traditional medicine, you can add certain herbal plants, for instance, turmeric or coconut oil, to your daily drink. This will not result in any abuse and no side effects. Also, some traditional practices do not involve ingesting medicinal plants.

Sometimes it is just inhaling with meditation, burning of a certain plant to purify the air, and several other practices that cannot resolve bodily damage. So, this can be easily incorporated into modern-day life. Like I said earlier, please do research on any medicinal plant you consume to know how much and how long you should consume this plant. Apart from this, traditional medicine also covers acupuncture, home therapy, and bone resetting. Meditation, for instance, can be incorporated into or daily or weekly exercise for wholeness.

CHAPTER THREE: ROLE OF NATIVE AMERICAN HEALING TRADITIONS

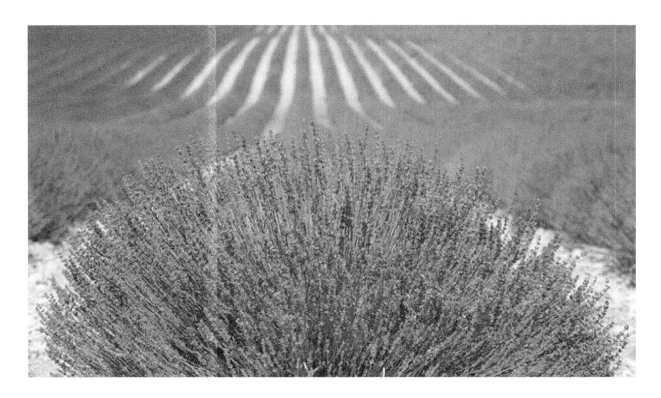

Traditional medicine has played a huge role in medicine as we know it today. Most of the plants and medication we have today were developed from the traditional practices of the Native American people. A lot of today's medications, like aspirin, came as a result of a test run on plants the Native Americans had used for hundreds of years to cure diseases. Although we now have these herbal properties chemically produced, we understand that it would have been impossible to have modern medicine as it is today without traditional medicine and the knowledge of the Native American people.

Recently people are beginning to see the link between wholeness of mind and the physical state of the body. It has been scientifically proven that the state of mind can cause some kinds of ailments like ulcers and other diseases. This is a new scientific Discovery but has been known to the traditional people for hundreds of years, hence the need to achieve total wholeness and not just healing of a particular element. Science seems to see ailments as individualistic and unique; traditional medicine considers them as a problem in mind and in the body.

This method of healing is more productive and more effective in stopping the disease from recurring. The role of traditional medicine is vast, and even though credit is not always given to it, it is the bedrock of our modern medicine today. Full patient-centered care can only be achieved by combining traditional and modern medicine to gain their individual holistic health needs.

Herbs That Have Played a Huge Role in American Medicine

1. ALLSPICE

Allspice has been used for hundreds of years to cure diseases and fight bacteria in the body. Allspice is especially used to kill bacteria in food. It is used for indigestion, intestinal gas, stomach pain, menstrual cramps, high blood pressure, diabetes, obesity, fever, the common cold and other diseases. Its aromatic compounds which are the polyphenols and glycosides also have antibacterial, antineuralgic and analgesic properties. Allspice happens to be one of those herbs that can kill almost all bacteria in food. Because of its antibacterial compounds, allspice protects the body by preventing E coli bacteria and yeast infection. Allspice can be added to meals or applied to the body topically to kill bacteria. It can also be ingested. The antioxidant in allspice prevents sugar from being stored in excess amounts in the body which in turn prevents diabetes and other sugar related diseases.

2. ANGELICA

Angelica is a medicinal plant that is used mostly for heartburn, loss of appetite, intestinal gas, arthritis, rheumatism, blood circulation problems, respiratory tract infections, cancer, insomnia, nervousness, anxiety and depression.

Angelica has antioxidants, anti-inflammatory and anti-bacterial properties which prevents bacterial infections in the body. It also promotes hair growth. Some people believe Angelica to be an abortifacient and have used this to cause an abortion. Angelica has also been said to cure brain cancer by killing glioblastoma cells. Angelica is often used for women's health including menopausal symptoms like hot flashes or night sweats. Using Angelica can reduce the intensity of these hot flashes. It is also used to relieve pains like rheumatism, muscle pains and other pains in the body.

3. ANISE

Anise is a popular herb. This plant is used to make medicine. The roots and the leaves of the herb are used for intestinal gas, stomach ache, cough, as appetite stimulants, and as a diuretic to increase the expulsion of fluids from the body. It has a lot of nutrients and that is where its health benefits are the same. This plant has antifungal, antibacterial and anti-inflammatory properties.

These properties help anise fight against bacteria in the body. It has the capacity to calm the digestive system and that is why this plant is still used today especially for children. It is also used as an antiseptic to treat cough, asthma and bronchitis. Anise also has sedative properties so it is used to treat mild insomnia. Its oil is also used to provide relief from rheumatism, back pain and to treat other symptoms that may be preventing a good night's rest.

4. ASAFOETIDA

Asafoetida is a medicinal plant that is used to treat whooping cough, asthma, flatulence, bronchitis, stomach ache, ulcer, epilepsy, stomach, parasite, digestion problems and the common cold. This plant is also used for stomach diseases. It has antibacterial, antifungal, and antimicrobial effects on the body so it doesn't just work for the stomach it also reduces blood pressure.

Asafoetida prevents cancer, protects the brain from developing certain diseases, relieves asthma and lower blood sugar levels which leads to prevention of hypertension. Science has confirmed that the chemicals in this plant relieves irritable bowel syndrome and protects against high blood pressure by reducing cholesterol and triglycerides in the body. It also has the capacity to feel blood in the veins which helps prevent high blood pressure. Because asafoetida improves metabolism it also helps burn calories which leads to weight loss. To harness the maximum benefits of this plant, get its powder and add it to your meals or make it a fertility drink first thing in the morning.

5. BERGAMOT

Science has confirmed that bergamot has medicinal uses. Bergamot induces sweating, reduces fever, helps in digestion, minimises cold, stops headache, relieves gastric disorders, helps manage nausea and also nourishes the skin. It has been used as a stimulant, as a relaxant and as a medication against colic. It reduces cholesterol and increases the good HDL cholesterol in the body.

Bergamot plant is generally safe for people though it may come with some side effects like dizziness or heartburn for some people. If you notice any reaction to this herb, stop taking it and ask for your doctor's counsel. This plant is calming so it reduces stress and anxiety and also allows for a good night rest. Use this herb to achieve better sleep and improve rest. You can take bergamot as a tea just before bedtime to help you sleep.

6. BLACK CUMIN

Black cumin is a seed that has a lot of medicinal benefits. It is used for chronic back pain, sinus infection, upper respiratory tract infections, cold, fever, cough and other infections. It can also be used for diabetes, paralysis, inflammation of the body, hypertension and digestive tract problems. It is also helpful in nourishing a healthy kidney and prevention of kidney inflammation. This herb also helps with penile dysfunction as it allows blood circulation to the genitals. The seed is generally safe for people but if you notice some side effects as usual speak with your doctor for guidance.

7. BLACK PEPPER

Black pepper is usually taken for asthma, bronchitis, arthritis, stomach problems, e colic depression, cholera, gas, headache, sexual libido, menstrual cramps, runny nose, sinus infection, dizziness, vitiligo, weight loss, cancer and discolored skin. Here are some of the benefits of black pepper that have been confirmed by scientific research: black pepper is high in antioxidant content. This means that black pepper fights harmful radicals in the body and rids the body of dangerous toxins that would have infected the body with diseases.

It has anti-inflammatory properties so it fights diseases in the tummy and other parts of the body. Black pepper also balances blood sugar levels by reducing high sugar content in the blood. Black pepper fights cancer in the body and lowers cholesterol levels which leads to prevention of hypertension. Black pepper boosts the immune system. It does this by boosting the white blood cells which the body uses to fight illnesses. Black pepper can be mixed with turmeric to obtain the maximum effect of the curcumin in turmeric. Black pepper is also good for colds as it decongests the windpipe and reduces the sneezing reflex.

8. CHIVES

Chives is a medicinal plant that is known to prevent cancer. Several scientific studies have shown that chives can prevent, slow down the progression or eliminate cancer. Chives also improve memory because they contain choline and folate. This property helps in memory improvement. Chives has vitamin k that helps to build bone density. Chives also have vitamin c which prevents some diseases by boosting the immune system. Chives also has a high content of vitamin A, beta carotene and iron which helps maintain a balanced blood pressure and increase immune system power.

9. CAYENNE PEPPER

Cayenne pepper has a lot of medicinal benefits. It helps with digestion, reduces headache, relieves migraine, detoxifies the system, relieves joint pains, helps with nausea and morning sickness, boosts metabolism which in turn helps with weight loss. It also relieves pain in joints and muscles.

Cayenne pepper has a high amount of antioxidants which helps flush out toxins and free radicals from the body. The capsaicin in cayenne pepper boosts metabolism by increasing body heat. This converts the food into energy therefore burning calories.

Cayenne, like other hot peppers, is especially good for burning belly fat. This pepper is also anti-inflammatory so it can be used to reduce or eliminate inflammation in the body. Cayenne heat can cause quick digestion and reduces constipation as a result.

10. POPPY SEEDS

Poppy seeds have a lot of health benefits. It aids in digestion, promotes healthier skin and can treat upper respiratory tract problems. Poppy seeds have high fibrous content so it helps in weight loss and prevents colon cancer. The fiber content also helps in constipation and digestion. Poppy seeds relax smooth muscles so it can be used to minimize menstrual cramps. Poppy seeds can also be used as a sedative for better night rest.

11. BURNET

Burnet is mainly used for ulcer, colitis, uterine tract infection, diarrhea, blood vessel issues, heavy menstrual flow, menopausal symptoms, irregular menstruation, menstrual cramps and other feminine problems. Burnet can be eaten as salad or drink as a juice. You can use burnet for indigestion problems, constipation and other abdominal problems.

12. CARAWAY

Caraway is mostly used for bloating, intestinal gas, loss of appetite, stomach and intestinal pains, digestive issues, cough, muscle congestion, uterine tract infection, constipation and other diseases. The seeds of caraway promote weight loss and digestive tract function. Caraway seeds can also reduce inflammation as it has anti-inflammatory properties. It also helps in expelling gas from the body. It can also be used for heartburn as it has a soothing effect. The seeds can be eaten on its own or added to other foods.

13. CHERVIL

Chervil is a medicinal plant. This plant helps in fluid retention, digestion issues, digestive tract health, high blood pressure, cough, common cold, fever and skin diseases. This plant is also used as a diuretic as it helps in fluid expulsion from the body. It is great for the kidney as it flushes out fluids and excess sodium. This plant can dissolve and expel kidney stones. It also prevents the formation of kidney stones. You can add this to meals to get results or make it as a drink. Take this first thing in the morning on an empty stomach or at least 20 minutes before meals to help with digestion problems.

14. SESAME

Now to the amazing sesame. Sesame has a high fiber content so it helps in weight loss digestion, prevents cancer of the colon, helps in passing out of food and prevents constipation. Sesame lowers bad cholesterol in the body and also reduces inflammation as it has anti-inflammatory properties. Sesame has vitamin b which helps the body fight against diseases. It lowers blood pressure and prevents hypertension. It also manages high blood pressure. This plant is also a good source of energy and healthy fats. Sesame contains iron, calcium and Omega 6. Sesame can be added to meals or grounded and prepared as a drink.

15. SORREL

Sorrel has high anti-inflammatory compounds so it can be used to reduce swelling, relieve pain, decongest the nasal passage and treat respiratory tract infections. This plant also helps flush excess sodium and toxins out of the kidney. This means that sorrel helps with kidney health. It also improves eyesight as it has properties that help with vision.

The plant regulates blood pressure and prevents development of hypertension. It is rich in fiber so it reduces constipation, bloating and diarrhea. Sorrel also reduces cholesterol in the body which manages heart conditions and reduce chances of heart attacks. Because of its high vitamin A content, it has been said to prevent cataract in the eye and help with vision improvement. This plant also helps boost immunity because of its high vitamin C content. It helps the body fight against harmful toxins and free radicals that would have affected the skin.

This plant is used mainly for skin conditions as it treats ringworm, eczema and other skin irritation. Sorrel can be added to salad and other foods. You can also blend and drink sorrel first thing in the morning on an empty stomach for maximum effect. Because of its work in the digestive system, sorrel can also be taken 20 minutes before a meal to help with the digestion of that meal.

CHAPTER FOUR: HOW MODERN RESEARCH CONFIRMS WHAT THE TRIBES HAVE KNOWN FOR MILLENNIA

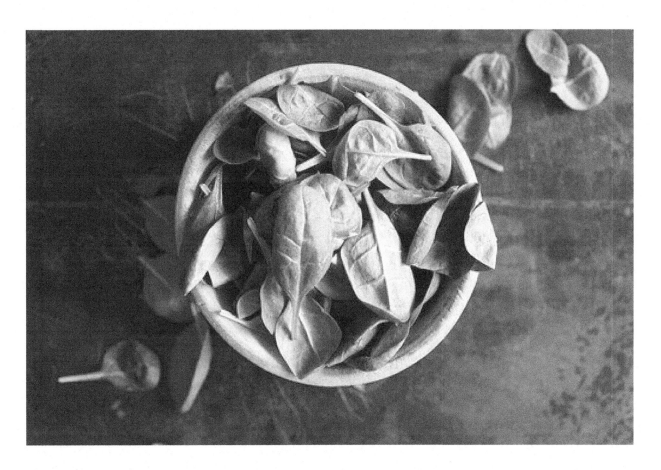

Modern research has confirmed a lot of what the Native American tribes knew about medicine. For instance, in aspirin production. The first aspirin was made from herbal plants that the Native Americans had been using as a pain reliever for hundreds of years.

Another is the belief in holistic healing that the Native Americans practice. It has been shown that some diseases are not physical and are caused by psychological or mental disorders. As earlier mentioned, it has been seen that physiological stress can alter the **PH Balance** in the body and cause ulcers, so the Native Americans were right when they said healing had to cover the mind, soul, environment, and body.

These are two of the many examples that science confirms Native American healing practices. Most of the medication we have today came through research of science on plants that were used by Native Americans. As it stands right now, plant-based medication makes up about 10% of medication produced worldwide, and most of these plants are used today because the Native Americans use them to cure their diseases.

So, it can be seen that although Native Americans did not use scientific equipment and technology to make their herbal medication more effective, they knew what they were doing, and they were right about most of the medication they were administered.

Herbs Used for Modern Medicine

1. TARRAGON

Tarragon is used to stimulate appetite, reduce nausea, toothache, insomnia and other conditions. Tarragon has a lot of health benefits. It reduces blood sugar inflammation and pain. This is due to the fact that tarragon has anti-inflammatory antioxidant and antifungal properties. It also purges the body of harmful toxins and free radicals that could harm the body. Tarragon also keeps the body in shape and prevents diseases. Tarragon can be eaten raw or added to meals. Tarragon is a diuretic as it allows the free flow of urine from the body.

2. WASABI

Wasabi is a medicinal plant that has antimicrobial, anti-inflammatory and antibacterial properties. Wasabi also has anti-cancer properties which prevents and fights cancer in the human body. Wasabi can kill a lot of viruses and bacteria like E coli, cholera and salmonella. Wasabi is good for the stomach as it is an antimicrobial agent that fights against some bacteria in the stomach. It also clears nasal congestion and heals sinus infections.

3. NUTMEG

Nutmeg has a lot of health benefits. It helps with indigestion, detoxifies the body of harmful toxins, helps with the production of collagen which positively affects the skin, reduces insomnia, boosts the immune system, lowers blood sugar and improves blood circulation.

Nutmeg has anti-inflammatory and antioxidant properties which make this nutmeg control blood sugar, improve moods, fight depression, and reduce anxiety. Nutmeg helps manage hypertension as it is rich in magnesium, potassium and calcium which lowers blood pressure. Nutmeg can be used to lighten the skin. Simply mix nutmeg powder with a teaspoon of lemon and a teaspoon of honey in a bowl. Put this on your face as a facial mask for 20 minutes. Wash off and dry the face with a towel. Nutmeg helps in relaxation by affecting the nervous system. If you are having trouble sleeping, grate nutmeg and mix with a glass of milk for improved quality of sleep.

4. LOVAGE

The lovage plant is best known for stomach discomfort. It is also used to help the upper respiratory system and treat heart conditions. It is essential for the body as it tackles kidney stones and excess sodium in the body.

This plant has been used to make medicine for inflammation and prevention of kidney stones. It also helps with urine or fluid retention in the body. This diuretic flushes the body with little or no side effects.

5. CILANTRO

Cilantro has an antimicrobial compound that protects the body from illness caused by tempered food. This means that when you consume food that has food poisoning, cilantro can help your body fight against the poisoning. This herb is also used to make medicine for cancer, measles, toothache and other conditions. Cilantro reduces the risk of heart disease, obesity, epilepsy and other diseases.

6. COSTMARY

The costmary plant is used to ease pains and menstrual cramps. It is also used to treat cough, cold, catarrh and muscle cramps. You can add this herb in your salad or other foods. You can also use it as a drink for pains and flu infections.

7. CORIANDER

Coriander plant is used mainly for stomach pain, constipation, diarrhea, nausea, intestinal gas and other conditions. This plant lowers blood sugar, helps improve the heart functions, promotes a well-balanced sugar levels, boosts the immune system, protects the brain and allows for the production of collagen which gives the skin a youthful glow. Coriander is anti-inflammatory that is why it can also be used for inflammatory diseases like arthritis. Coriander is especially good for the kidney because of its phosphorus, calcium, and potassium properties. This improves digestion and kidney functions. Coriander relaxes blood vessels; this helps prevent high blood pressure.

8. PARSLEY

The parsley leaf seed and root have been used to make medicine for many years. People mainly use parsley for kidney stones, diabetes, asthma, high blood pressure, constipation, cough and uterine tract infections. Parsley cleanses the kidneys because it acts as a diuretic which flushes sodium and fluids out of the kidney.

It also prevents formation of kidney stones. Apart from that, it flushes kidney stones. Parsley has high nitrate content which helps the blood vessels relax. This protects the body against high blood pressure. Parsley can be taken as a juice in the morning to cleanse the system. Simply blend parsley, pour into a glass, add honey and drink as a smoothie.

9. HYSSOP

Hyssop plant is mainly used for digestive tract problems, liver and gallbladder problems, colic and loss of appetite. It can also be used for common cold, cough, sore throat, asthma and other respiratory tract problems. Hyssop can be taken as tea or added to meals. For best effect, add fresh hyssop to salad, pasta or other foods.

10. MARJORAM

Marjoram plant is mainly used to heal tooth ache, joint pains, digestive tract infections, asthma, indigestion, headache, rheumatism and hypertension. This plant is considered beneficial for the heart because it allows for better blood circulation. Which means that this plant prevents or manages high blood pressure in people. Marjoram can also be used for gallbladder disease, digestive problems, depression, paralysis and anxiety. It is also used to relax the muscles in the uterus which helps lower the pains of menstruation. It also cures insomnia as it has some sedative properties that deal with insomnia. You can add marjoram to your food or take it as a drink. You can also diffuse it in a diffuser for an improved night rest.

CHAPTER FIVE: HERBAL MEDICINE 101: HOW YOU CAN HARNESS THE POWER OF HEALING HERBS

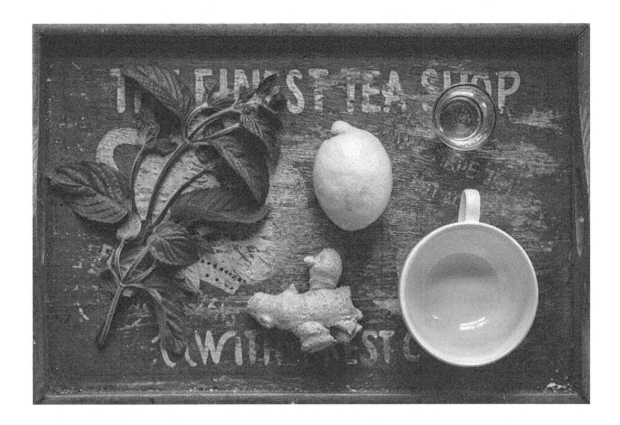

I personally believe that the best herbs one can get are the fresh ones right out of the garden. This means that the medicinal herb still has its moisture stuck inside the leaves which goes a long way in giving the body 100% benefits of the medicine contained in the plant. Also, there's no fear of adulteration or taking herbs from unknown sources. There is also the assurance a person gets from harvesting certain plants at the right time. You will know if the plants are organic or not. If you do not plant the herbs yourself, you can go to an organic market and buy them there.

Ways to get the best out of medicinal plants:

1. Ask Questions

Is this herb good for me?

We have to emphasize on this that medicinal plants may be generally good for people but not the best option for an individual. This is because everybody is different and what is good for one person may cause allergic reactions in another person. So, before you incorporate traditional medicine with modern medicine, do well to ask either the traditional medicine man or the modern physician about the herb you are about to take. Your personal history plus medical advice can go a long way to determine if a particular herb is good for your body system. If it is discovered that this herb is not good for you, no matter how effective it is in curing your ailment or the testimonies of others please desist from using it as it may cause you more harm than good. Even traditional healers always put the individual into consideration, that is why they do not have herbs made for mass consumption but take a look at every person to mix unique herbs for that particular person's need.

It is very unwise to take herbs without knowing if it is good for you. For instance, peanuts are a general meal for most Americans and people all around the world but it has been shown to adversely affect the thyroid functions. So, in that instance someone with goiter or other thyroid malfunctions would not be advised to take any traditional medicine that has peanuts. This too applies to other herbs. So, we could say turmeric is healthy and should be incorporated in meals but if for one reason or the other turmeric is not healthy for you, you would not get the benefit of turmeric but instead have to deal with the problems and side effects of taking turmeric with your health conditions. There are also some medicinal herbs that we've discussed in this book which help in thinning the blood. If you are battling hemorrhage it will be bad to take these herbs because they will cause bleeding. So, the first question to ask when anybody tells you of the effectiveness of a particular herb is to ask if this herb is good for you? This question will help you know what to take and what to avoid. What works for Mr. A may not work for Mr. B.

Will this herb interact with my medication?

Like we've already discussed in this book adequate research is needed to take any medicinal plant as this research will help you know if this herb can interact with your medication and render the medication ineffective or make it work in the opposite direction. Most of these herbs should not be taken with alcohol as alcohol can heighten its effects or lower the effect of the medication.

Always speak with a doctor to find out if the herb you are taking can interact with any dietary supplements you are on or if they can affect the effectiveness of the medication you have been placed on. This will help you make informed choices on the kind of herbs to avoid.

How long can I use this herb and what are its side effects?

No matter how good herbs are they have to be used for a certain period of time and after the period of time they should be stopped. This is because they are medicinal and prolonged use could result in some problems. Always know how long you can use the herbs and how long it will take for you to see results so that you don't use it for a very short while and think that the herb was not effective in curing your problem. Traditional herbs are not like modern medicine; they take longer periods to work because their potency have not been heightened in laboratories, so they don't work as fast as the laboratory produced medication. Therefore, traditional herbs take a longer period in showing results, so when taking herbs, you have to bear in mind that the results may be on the way.

Also note that each herb has its own time frame, so it can take a person one week to see results in a certain herb and it may take another person who uses a different herb a longer period to see results. The truth is each plant is different and unique and it also acts differently with different human beings. So, your friend may use Merrick and see results in a few days because of her body type and you use the same Merrick and not see results for a few weeks. You have to understand the different body types also affect how medicinal plants work.

Where are the herbs gotten from and how sustainable is the production?

The plant should be organic at least. Most people, because of how popular some medicinal plants are, have taken to planting them with the help of chemicals in order to get this plant ready for sale in the shortest period possible. These plants that are chemically cultivated have lesser potency than the ones that grow naturally in their natural habitat. Also, it is known that plant flourish better in their natural habitat than in controlled nurseries. The chemical contents are also different because the natural ones mostly come from natural roots or other sources that give it time to germinate, grow and flourish with all the nutritional and medicinal content taking its time to mature. But when they are taken out of their natural habitat some of this plant fails to grow as fast as the farmer would have wanted. This leads to all the chemical aid to assist the plants growth or to even achieve basic survival. The chemical method of planting rushes the plant to maturity but takes away the development of most of the natural nutrients of the plant. When these natural compounds are not present, the plant will look and feel like its natural counterpart but it's basically empty as it lacks the essential compounds that can be used in medicine.

Whether it is of the purest quality or it has been adulterated?

It is important to note if the herb is purely the plant or whether it has been adulterated. This can make a whole difference between getting well or getting worse. Out of greed, manufacturers of store sold herbs have decided to cheat people and make billions out of selling adulterated herbs. Some of the things added to these herbs are inedible and downright poisonous which can lead to grievous illnesses or even death. It is stated that a meaningful amount of oregano sold in the UK is adulterated with olive leaves and myrtle leaves. The same thing can be said for the sage plant. The only way to be sure that your herb is 100% pure is by planting them in your garden or buying from a reliable vendor.

2. Follow Instructions

Traditional medicine is different from modern medicine. A lot of people feel like they can actually abuse traditional plants and get away with it because there is little chemical content but that is not true. Traditional medicine can be abused. To get the best out of a plant and take the right dosage of the help, do not rush the medication or steer off course. Always take the medication when it should be taken consistently till the end.

Also, it will be more effective if taken at the same time every day. This is better than taking in the morning or the first day and in the evening of the second day as it will mess the cycle of 24 hours to maybe 36 hours and then back to 24 hours. If the herb is meant to be steamed then steaming cannot be replaced with diffusing. If it's meant to be taken as tea then it means it will be most potently taken as tea and not as a cold drink. Always follow instructions on how to use the different herbs.

If you do not feel better after taking the medication recommended, talk to your doctor and stop taking the medication.

3. Be Observant

No matter how much people praise a plant's efficacy, you still have to look at things for yourself and observe how your body reacts to the herb. It is best to be observant when treating an ailment with a medicinal plant because much research has not really been done on so many herbs. Therefore, individuals have to really rely on their own personal observations when taking traditional medicine. If your observation shows that you should stop taking the traditional medicine it will do you much good to desist from taking it. Also, if you observe that a particular dosage is not good for you, you could always readjust to one that favors your body system.

BOOK 2
HERBAL APOTHECARY
OF NATIVE AMERICA

CHAPTER ONE: PROFILE OF 100
HERBS AND WILD PLANTS

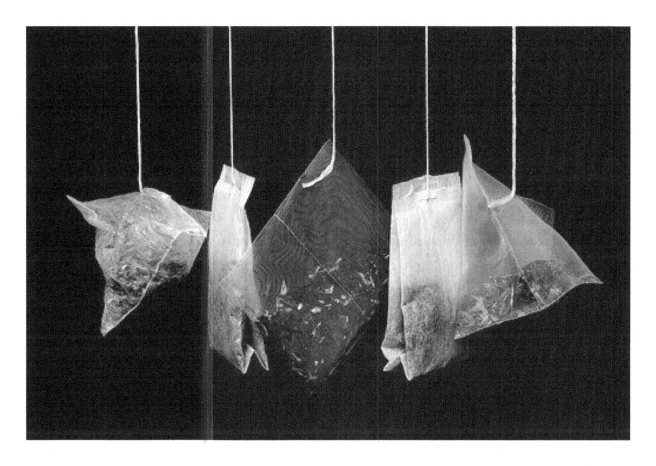

There are a lot of medicinal herbs and wild plants, most of which look so identical that they cannot be differentiated by most people. This leads to confusion and sometimes to the dangerous mistake of taking an inedible plant as a medicinal herb which can lead to serious diseases or even death.

Another reason why plants are profiled is because the plant should be classified according to their different families and species which could help people take note of the little differences between different species of the same family. Sometimes these little differences can be very important as they cure very different ailments. So, without profiling, someone could end up taking herb meant for one ailment for a totally different one which leads to an abuse of the medicine.

Listed below are the profiles of a hundred herbs and wild plants:

COFFEE

Scientific name: Coffea Arabica

Family: Rubiaceae (coffee madder)

DESCRIPTION

There are two main species which are cultivated commercially and they are: coffea canephora and c Arabica. C. canephora is mostly cultivated in the Western and Central Subsaharan Africa from Guinea to Uganda and Southern Sudan. C. Arabica is mostly cultivated in Latin America, Eastern Africa, Asia and Arabia.

FACTS

Coffee produces different blends of flavors. The type and blend of coffee beans, roasting method, preparation method and where it originates determines the kind of flavors it will produce. The aroma can be nutty, herby, flowery, or smoky. The taste can either be bitter, sweet, acidic or salty. The manner in which the coffee beans were roasted determines the kind of aroma it will produce.

NATURAL HABITAT

According to legends, coffee was first recognized for its energetic effect in Ethiopia by the Oromo people. Coffee beans were first roasted and brewed in Southern Arabia. Coffee plants are cultivated in 70 countries but are predominately cultivated in America, Southeast Asia, India and Africa. Brazil is currently the leading country that produces coffee seeds. Coffee was introduced into Europe in the 16th century. Until the 17th century, only Yemen supplied coffee; however, coffee was cultivated in America in the 18th century in Hawaiian Islands.

USES

Coffee contains caffeine which stimulates the central nervous system, muscles and heart. It boosts a person's physical performance because it increases the adrenaline in the body which improves mental alertness. It contains substances like: magnesium and potassium which regulate blood sugar levels. It breaks down the fat cells in the body, that is, it aids the burning of fat. Researchers have shown that coffee reduces premature death by 25%. It contains antioxidants which protect the body from free radicals that reside within it. It lowers the risk of Alzheimer disease by 65% and Parkinson's disease by 32 to 60%. It contains nutrients like: vitamin B2, vitamin B5 and vitamin B3. It also lowers the risk of Type 2 Diabetes by 20 to 53%. It protects the liver against diseases like hepatitis and fatty liver. It fights against depression and lowers the risk of cancer.

TRADITIONAL USES

Coffee is one of the most popular herbs in the world. It should be noted that coffee was used by the native Americans as a stimulant and medication for several ailments. Coffee was prepared traditionally by making a tea from its leaves and pounding its green seeds and was made into cakes. It was used to stimulate digestion and this is achieved by stimulating the release of gastric enzymes and increasing peristalsis. It was used to filter the kidney which increases urination. It mitigates the effect of metabolic diseases. It was used to relieve headaches.

GINGER

Scientific name: Zingider officinale

Family: Zingiberaceae

DESCRIPTION

Ginger is used as spice and is regarded as folk medicine. It grows annual pseudostems about one meter tall. It is a flowering plant that has pale yellow petals with purple edges. It is the roots that's used as spice.

NATURAL HABITAT

Ginger was first recorded in the Analects of Confucius. It originated from the tropical and subtropical forest of Southeast Asia. It was one of the spices that were exported from Asia. It was used by ancient Greeks and Romans. India is the leading producing country when it comes to ginger. It is native to humid and shaded habitants.

FACTS

Ginger is a rhizome. Rhizome is an underground stem. It is an herb. The Zingiberaceae family includes turmeric. Ginger is mostly harvested after 10 to 12 months. It also grows 4ft tall. It has a lot of health benefits.

USES

Ginger contains a lot of nutrients like: vitamin B3, vitamin B6, iron, potassium, vitamin C, magnesium, phosphorus, zinc, folate, riboflavin and niacin. It eases an upset stomach. It reduces inflammation and lowers blood sugar levels. It reduces the risk of cancer and relieves menstrual cramps. It can be used to prevent colds.

TRADITIONAL USES

It was used to alleviate colds. It is an ancient remedy in the Iranian traditional medicine. It was used as a tonic for memory, digestive system, expels compact wind from stomach and intestines and also used as aphrodisiac.

PARSLEY

Scientific name: Petroselinum crispum

Family:

DESCRIPTION

It is one of the most cultivated herbs in the world. It is a hardy plant and the leaves are triangular in shape with serrated edges. The plant blooms in its second year. The flowers are small and either green or yellow in color.

NATURAL HABITAT

It originated from the Mediterranean region. It grows well in a moist area. It can be grown outdoors or indoors.

FACTS

It is aromatic and it adds flavor to food. It can be used to garnish and decorate dishes.

USES

TRADITIONAL USES

OREGANO

Scientific name: Origanum vulgare

Family: Lamiaceae

DESCRIPTION

The plant grows up to 3 ft tall. The flower is pink – lilac in color. It has sturdy square stems. It blooms during summer.

NATURAL HABITAT

It originated from Africa and mild regions in Europe. It grows well where the climate is warm.

FACTS

It is predominately used in Greek and Italian dishes. It can be used either fresh or dried. It needs low water to survive. As a result of the many glands that the leaves have, it provides a strong scent when crushed. Essential oil like carvacrol and thymol can be gotten from oregano.

USES

It provides antioxidants which helps the body to eliminate free radicals. It contains anti – inflammatory properties which can reduce inflammation that could lead to autoimmune arthritis, allergic asthma and rheumatoid arthritis. It has anti – cancer properties. It can help to manage type 2 diabetes. It has a lot of health benefits.

BASIL

Scientific name: Ocimum basilicum

Family: Lamiaceae

DESCRIPTION

The flowers are small and dainty. It is white or dark purple in color. It grows from seed. It can be grown indoors or outdoors. It grows up to 24 inches in height.

NATURAL HABITAT

It originated from Africa and Asia. It grows well where the temperatures are mild. It strives where the sun is full and the soil must be moist. It is native to tropical regions.

FACTS

It is one of the most cultivated herbs in the world. It is grown annually. It is used to cook and garnish dishes. The herb can be used as fresh or dried.

USES

It is antibacterial, antiviral, antifungal, anti – inflammatory and analgesic. It must heal faster. It can be used against infections like mouth ulcers, keloids, raised scars and acne. It lowers blood sugar and cholesterol levels. It eases joint pain and protects the stomach.

THYME

Scientific name: Thymus vulgaris

Family: Lamiaceae

DESCRIPTION

It is a culinary herb. It grows well in dry and sandy soils. It grows up to 1 ft tall. It is either white or purple in color.

NATURAL HABITAT

It is native of Mediterranean region. It was first cultivated by the Ancient Egyptians. It is native to hot and sunny regions with well-drained soil. It grows on mountain highlands and dry slopes.

FACTS

It was used during European Middle Ages to aid sleep and prevent nightmares. It was used as incense. It was believed to bring courage. It can be used fresh or dried.

USES

It contains components like linalool, carvacrol, a- terpineol and cineole. It has antioxidant properties. The essential oil which is referred to as thymol found in thyme contains the following compounds: p cymene, myrcene, linalool and borneol. It can be used to reduce blood pressure. It has anti- cancer properties. It can be used to treat yeast infection, acne and skin problems.

ROSEMARY

Scientific name: Rosmarinus officinalis

Family: Lamiaceae

DESCRIPTION

It can grow up to 2 ft tall. The leaves are narrow and needle – shaped.

NATURAL HABITAT

It is native to Mediterranean region. It can thrive in extreme climate conditions. It also grows on rocky cliffs and dry scrub.

FACTS

It is a perennial plant. The flower is either light blue, pale violet, white or pink in color. It has long protruding stamens. It can be crushed and turned to powder.

USES

It is an herb and known for its essential oil which stimulates blood circulation. The oil is an essential ingredient in body oils, creams, perfumes and ointments. It is a good source of calcium, iron and vitamin B. It eases muscle pain, boosts the immune and circulatory system, hair growth, improves digestion and improves memory.

CASCARA SAGRADA

Scientific name: cascara buckthorn

Family: Rhamnus purshiana

DESCRIPTION

The dried bark is used as medicine. It is a stimulant laxative. It is sometimes referred to as bitter tonic

FACTS

It is prepared in both liquid and solid forms. The bitter less extract of the herb can be used as a flavoring agent.

NATURAL HABITAT

It is cultivated in North America and Kenya. It grows on the lower portion of mountains in the forests of the Pacific Northwest.

USES

It is used as a laxative because it contains a substance called anthraquinones. It is used to treat constipation. It can be used as a supplement. It lowers potassium in the body.

GINSENG

Scientific name: Panax ginseng

Family: Araliaceae

DESCRIPTION

It is a stimulating tea. They are perennial herbs. It is bisexual plant. It requires 5 to 7 years to mature from seed.

FACTS

It is a medicinal herb. It should not be used for more than two months. It is aromatic. It is used by Chinese as a panacea for illnesses.

NATURAL HABITAT

It is originated from Asia and native to Eastern North American, and grows in deciduous and mixed forests in the northeast of the United States of America and Canadian provinces of Quebec and Ontario.

USES

The roots have a lot of health benefits like: lowering the blood sugar levels and cholesterol levels. It is used to treat erectile dysfunction. It helps to calm nerves and alleviate depression. It boosts metabolism in the body. It improves sexual performance, learning and memory.

GARLIC

Scientific name: allium sativum

Family: Amaryllidaceae

DESCRIPTION

It is a perennial herb that grows from a bulb. It grows up to 3ft. The flower can either be pink or purple in color. The bulb contains 12 to 20 cloves.

FACTS

It has antibacterial, antiseptic and antifungal agents. It has compounds like zinc and sulphur which makes sleeping easier. It can be used as an appetite suppressant.

NATURAL HABITAT

It originated from Central Asia. It is cultivated in a warm, moderate climate.

USES

It is used to normalize blood pressure and reduce sugar levels and cholesterol levels. It is used to cure colds and flu. It fights against cancer cells. It is used to treat yeast infection.

GINKGO

Scientific name: Ginkgo biloba

Family: Ginkgoaceae

DESCRIPTION

It is also called a maidenhair tree. It is about 66 to 115 ft tall and 8 ft in diameter. It is deeply rooted and resistant to wind and snow damage. The branches are angular and long.

FACTS

It was discovered over 290 million years ago. It is a widely cultivated plant. The leaves turn to yellow and fall within 1 to 15 days during autumn. It is insect and fungus resistant. It can live up to 2,500 years old. It is referred to as a living fossil.

NATURAL HABITAT

It is native to China and the Northern Hemisphere. It was planted in ancient Chinese and Japanese temple gardens.

USES

It is a traditional Chinese medicine. It is used to treat Alzheimer disease because of its memory enhancing properties. The plant nut can be roasted and it is a delicacy in some regions. It is used to prepare damaged tissues. It can be used to reduce inflammation in arthritis, cancer, heart disease and stroke. It can increase blood flow. It improves brain function and reduces anxiety.

ABRONIA FRAGRANS

Scientific name: Sunan kimiyya

Family: Nyctaginaceae

DESCRIPTION

It is about 8 to 40 inches tall. The flowers consist of 4 to 5 petaloid sepals and sepaloid bracts with a tubular corolla borne in clusters of 25 to 80 at the ends of stems.

FACT

It is aromatic. The flowers of this plant open in the evening and close in the morning, a habit which gives the Nyctaginaceae family the common name of Four O'clocks

NATURAL HABITAT

It grows in sandy, loose and dry soils, plains and pastures. It is native to Northern Arizona, Western Texas, Oklahoma, Chihuahua and Mexico.

USES

It has many health benefits and treats some ailments. It is used to treat stomach ache, insect bite, mouth and cold sores. It has antibacterial properties which prevents wounds from getting infected when used to wash it. It is an antidote for swallowing spiders.

DOUGLAS MAPLE

Scientific name: Acer glabrum

Family: Sapindaceae

DESCRIPTION

It is about 33 ft tall with broad leaves. The flowers are yellowish – green in color.

FACT

It is a medicinal herb. The foliage is browsed by cattle, sheep and game animals.

NATURAL HABITAT

It is native to Alaska South, Washington and Idaho.

USES

It increases production of breast milk in nursing mothers. It is used to treat diarrhea and swelling.

BOX ELDER

Scientific name: Acer negundo

Family: Sapindaceae

DESCRIPTION

It has a lifespan of 60 years. It is about 35 to 80 ft tall with a diameter of about 3.3 ft.

FACT

It was used as incense to cleanse the environment. It can be cooked or eaten raw. It is used to make beverages and candies. It has a lot of medicinal benefits.

NATURAL HABITAT

It is native to the United States and Canada.

USES

It is used to induce vomiting. It can be used for respiratory diseases, wounds, paralysis and swelling. The leaves of the plant can be used to preserve vegetables and fruits.

SILVER MAPLE

Scientific name: Acer saccharinum

Family: Sapindaceae

DESCRIPTION

It can grow to be about 35 meters tall with a trunk that is more than 100 centimeters in diameter. The leaves are 15 to 20 centimeters long.

FACT

It is sometimes planted to provide shade and it grows quickly.

NATURAL HABITAT

It is native to America.

USES

It is used to treat dysentery and cramps. It alleviates soreness in the body. It is an effective medicine for women.

BLACK COHOSH

Scientific name: Actaea racemosa

Family: Ranunculaceae

DESCRIPTION

This wildflower has small plumes of star-shaped white flowers that reach up to 8 feet and more commonly 4 to 6 feet tall above deep green, fern-like leaves.

NATURAL HABITAT

It is native to North America.

USES

It is used to relieve menopausal symptoms in women. It is used to treat vertigo, anxiety, stress, irritation, tinnitus, nervousness, vaginal dryness, hot flashes and heart palpitations. It is used to insomnia. It is used to regulate the menstrual cycle, shed the uterine lining and tone the uterus.

TALL HAIRY AGRIMONY

Scientific name: Agrimonia gryposepala

Family: Rosaceae

DESCRIPTION

It is a medicinal herb.

FACT

The flowers are ¼ to about 1/3 inch across with 5 oval yellow petals and 5 to 10 yellow stamens, the tips yellow to orange. Alternating with the petals are 5 green sepals that are pointed at the tip, sparsely hairy and slightly shorter than the petals.

NATURAL HABITAT

It grows well where the dry soil is moist, open woods, woodland edges, thickets, fields, banks and swamps. It is native North America.

USES

It is used to stop bleeding, treat gastric problems, uterine tract infection, fever, liver infection, stomach flu, irritable bowel syndrome, cough, sore throat, eczema, tuberculosis, bladder leakage, cancer, gall bladder disorder, insomnia, diabetes, cancer and diarrhea. It reduces heavy menstrual flow.

RAMP

Scientific name: Allium tricoccum

Family: Amaryllidaceae

DESCRIPTION

It produces a cluster of 2–6 bulbs that give rise to broad, flat, smooth, light green leaves that are 20–30 cm long including the narrow petioles, with deep purple or burgundy tints on the lower stems.

FACT

The leaves are edible. It is a perennial plant.

NATURAL HABITAT

It is native to North America.

USES

It is rich in selenium, calcium and vitamins. It improves eyesight, boosts the immune and cardiovascular system. It cleanses the body of harmful toxins and radicals. It is used to treat digestive system, inflammation, liver problem, heart diseases, hypertension and cancer. It has antibacterial properties.

WHITE ALDER

Scientific name: Alnus rhombifolia

Family: Betulaceae

DESCRIPTION

It grows up to 9-82 ft and rarely up to 115 ft tall, with pale gray bark, smooth on young trees, becoming scaly on old trees. The leaves are alternate, rhombic to narrow elliptic, long and broad, with a finely serrated margin and a rounded to acute apex

FACT

It can tolerate infertile soils.

NATURAL HABITAT

It is native to North America. It grows well in riparian zone habitat.

USES

It is used to treat different ailments, especially the female reproductive system. It is used to treat inflammation, fever, ovarian and breast cancer, menstruation and lactation. The plant bark can be used to make balm which is used to treat skin problems like eczema, burns, wounds, hemorrhoids and ringworm.

RED ALDER

Scientific name: Alnus rubra

Family: Betulaceae

DESCRIPTION

It is about 66 to 98 ft tall. The leaves are ovate and 7 to 15 centimeters long, with bluntly serrated edges

FACT

It is red in color. The name is derived from the red color that develops when the bark is bruised or scraped.

NATURAL HABITAT

It is native to Western North America.

USES

It is used to treat cancer, poison, insect bite and tuberculosis.

THE CALIFORNIA SAGEBRUSH

Scientific name: Artemisia californica

Family: Asteraceae

DESCRIPTION

It grows from the base and up to 8 ft tall. The stems are flexible, hairless and fuzzy. The leaves are about 10 centimeters long and the color is light green.

FACT

It is a fact that sage can be used in cooking and spice and infused in hot water to make tea.

NATURAL HABITAT

It is native to some regions in North America.

USES

It is used to treat heavy bleeding, menopausal symptoms like hot flashes and night sweating. It is also used to treat cramps, and induce labor. Apart from these feminine ailments, it is effective for cough, sore throat, fever, pain reliever, mouth sores, insect bites, uterine tract infections, bronchitis and sinus infections.

CALIFORNIA MUGWORT

Scientific name: Artemisia douglasiana

Family: Asteraceae

DESCRIPTION

It is a perennial herb and it grows from a colony of rhizomes. It is about 1.6 to 8.2 ft tall.

FACT

It is anti-inflammatory, anti-tumor, antifungal, anticoagulant and antidiabetic. It blooms between May and October.

NATURAL HABITAT

It grows well in coarse soils. It is native to Western United States.

USES

It is used to prevent pregnancies. It is used to treat arthritis, insect bite, headache, chest pain, rashes, bruises, joints, rheumatism, mild insomnia, irregular periods, hysteria, convulsion, epilepsy, blood circulation and stimulate gastric gases. It hydrates skin and nourishes hair. As an antitumor, it can be used to fight against some kinds of cancer.

WHITE SAGEBRUSH

Scientific name: Artemisia ludoviciana

Family: Asteraceae

DESCRIPTION

It is a rhizomatous perennial plant growing about 1.1 to 3.3 ft tall. The stems are either covered in woolly gray or white hairs.

FACT

It was used as protection against negative energies. It was used as incense and burned in native American religious rituals.

NATURAL HABITAT

It is native to North America.

USES

It is used to treat skin problems, cold, fever, cough, indigestion and diarrhea. It relieves cramps and lowers cholesterol and sugar levels.

GIANT CANE

Scientific name: Arundinaria gigantea

Family: Poaceae

DESCRIPTION

It is a perennial grass that is rounded and the stem is 7 cm in diameter and it is about 33 ft tall. The leaves are 30 cm long and 4 cm wide.

FACTS

It is a flood plant for southern pearly eye and butterfly.

NATURAL HABITAT

It is native to America. It grows well in monotypic colonies and pine forest.

USES

It is used to treat ulcer, gastritis, headache, muscle pain, diseases in the liver, respiratory and digestive system.

CANADA WILD GINGER

Scientific name: Asarum canadense

Family: Aristolochiaceae

DESCRIPTION

The leaves are kidney shaped. It blooms from April to June. The flowers are hairy.

FACTS

It contains components like aristolochic acid and is carcinogenic and it can cause kidney damage.

NATURAL HABITAT

It is native to Eastern North America and grows well in deciduous forest.

USES

It is used to add flavor and season food. It treats ailments like fever, cramps, asthma, convulsions, urinary disorders, swollen breasts, sexually transmitted diseases, indigestion, colic, stomach ache, digestive and upper respiratory system problems.

WHORLED MILKWEED

Scientific name: Asclepias verticillata

Family: Apocynaceae

DESCRIPTION

It is a perennial plant and about 2.5 ft tall. It has unbranched stems which are long, narrow, sessile and needle-like.

FACTS

It reproduces vegetatively. It is a host for monarch butterflies and is toxic to livestock.

NATURAL HABITAT

It is native to Eastern North America and Western Canada.

USES

It is used to treat snake bite, lung diseases, diarrhea, rheumatism, pleurisy, asthma, fever, rashes, swelling and respiratory tract problems.

DESERT BROOM

Scientific name: Baccharis sarothroides

Family: Asteraceae

DESCRIPTION

The leaves are small and thick.

FACTS

It has anti – inflammatory, antifungal and antioxidants properties.

NATURAL HABITAT

It is native to North America. It grows in gravelly dry soils.

USES

It is used to treat headaches, body aches, joint pains, colic, arthritis, sinus infections, sore throat and rheumatism. It reduces cholesterol levels in the body.

ARROWLEAF BALSAMROOT

Scientific name: Balsamorhiza sagittata

Family: Asteraceae

DESCRIPTION

It is about 20 to 60 cm tall.

FACTS

It is medicinal and used to cook.

NATURAL HABITAT

It is native to North America.

USES

It is used to treat wounds, bruises, cough, cold, fever and tuberculosis.

EVENING PRIMROSE

Scientific name: Oenothera

Family: Onagraceae

DESCRIPTION

The flower is yellow in color.

FACTS

It is a species of Oenothera biennis.

NATURAL HABITAT

It is native to North America and Europe.

USES

It is used to treat skin problems, arthritis, menopause symptoms, asthma, chronic fatigue, pregnancy complication, rheumatism, arthritis, cancer, cold, acne, heart disease, ulcerative colitis, dementia, hot flashes, vaginal dryness, inflammation, prostaglandins and infertility problems.

DEVIL'S CLUB

Scientific name: Oplopanax horridus

Family: Araliaceae

DESCRIPTION

It is about 3 to 4 ft tall.

FACTS

It is known for its large leaves and woody stems.

NATURAL HABITAT

It is native to North America.

USES

It is used to treat fever, stomach ache, tuberculosis, cancer, stomach ache, cough, diabetes, low blood sugar, pneumonia, sore throat, eczema, skin problems, wounds, inflammation, rheumatism and arthritis.

ECHINACEA

Scientific name: Echinacea purpurea

Family: Asteraceae

DESCRIPTION

It is about 120 cm tall and 25 cm wide.

FACTS

It has 10 different species. It has been used for hundreds of years.

NATURAL HABITAT

It is native to Eastern and Central North America.

USES

It boosts the immune system and fights infections and viruses. It is used to treat cold, fever, flu, pain reliever, respiratory problems, wound and high blood pressure.

GOLDENSEAL

Scientific name: Hydrastis canadensis

Family: Ranunculaceae

DESCRIPTION

It is a thick yellow knitted rootstock plant.

FACTS

NATURAL HABITAT

It is native to North America.

USES

It is used to treat stomach ache, peptic ulcer, hemorrhoids, constipation, swelling, sinus infection, skin infections or disorders, cramps, heavy menstrual flow, sores, bruises and rashes. It removes blemishes and tones the skin.

GRAPE

Scientific name: Vitis vinifera

Family: Vitaceae

DESCRIPTION

It is a medicinal herb.

FACTS

NATURAL HABITAT

It is native to Mediterranean region, Central Europe and Southwestern Asia.

USES

It is used to flush out toxins from the body, repair skin, fight cancer and rejuvenate the skin. It is used to treat wrinkles, saggy skin, wounds, cardiovascular diseases, cancer and stretch marks.

CRANBERRY

Scientific name: Vaccinium subg oxycocus

Family: Ericaceae

DESCRIPTION

It is about 7ft long and 20cm in height.

FACTS

It contains nutrients like polyphenols which are good for the brain. It has antioxidant, anti – inflammatory, anti-fungal and anti-viral content.

NATURAL HABITAT

USES

It is used to boost immunity, constipation, treat urinary tract infection, hypertension, urinary tract, skin blemishes, rashes and scars. It's good for hair growth.

UMBELLATA

Scientific name: Ficus umbellata

Family: Apocynaceae

DESCRIPTION

The fruit is yellow and smooth.

FACTS

It was used as arrow poison.

NATURAL HABITAT

It is native to the rainforest region.

USES

It is used to treat bladder stones, prostatitis, cystitis, urinary tract infection, dehydration and aids weight loss.

TEA TREE

Scientific name: Melaleuca alternifolia

Family: Myrtaceae

DESCRIPTION

It grows up to 7ft tall.

FACTS

It has antibacterial, anti-viral and anti-inflammatory properties.

NATURAL HABITAT

It is native to Australia.

USES

It is used to treat eczema, dandruff, lice, inflammation, insect bite and eye infections. It repairs pores, smoothen skin and moisturize the skin.

FLAX SEED

Scientific name: Linum usitatissimum

Family: Linaceae

DESCRIPTION

It is about 3 ft tall.

FACTS

It is rich in Omega 3 fat, vitamin D and B.

NATURAL HABITAT

USES

It is used to treat high blood pressure, diarrhea, fertility issues, and heart diseases. It aids weight loss, lower cholesterol levels. It moisturizes and smoothens the skin. It regulates hormonal imbalances and menstruation.

CHIA SEED

Scientific name: salvia hispanica

Family: Lamiaceae

DESCRIPTION

It is an annual plant and 5 ft 9 in height.

FACTS

It has low calories.

NATURAL HABITAT

It is native to Central and Southern Mexico

USES

It aids weight loss and boosts the digestive system. It flushes out harmful toxins and free radicals.

ERIGENIA

Scientific name: Erigenia bulbosa

Family: Apiaceae

DESCRIPTION

It is 5 to 15 cm tall.

FACTS

It can be chewed and used to cook.

NATURAL HABITAT

It is native to North America.

USES

It is used to treat toothache by chewing on the plant.

YERBA SANTA

Scientific name: Eriodictyon californicum

Family: Boraginaceae

DESCRIPTION

It is 3 to 4 ft tall.

FACTS

It is a medicinal herb and used to cleanse the environment from bad energies.

NATURAL HABITAT

It is native to America.

USES

It is used to treat colds, migraines, headaches, muscle pain, arthritis, chronic bronchitis, cough, tuberculosis, asthma, fever, skin problems, digestive system problems and colds.

WHITE GOURD

Scientific name: Benincasa hispida

Family: Cucurbitoidaeae

DESCRIPTION

It is a vine grown for its large fruit.

FACTS

It contains protein, vitamins, carotene, flavonoids and sucrose.

NATURAL HABITAT

It is native to Asia.

USES

It detoxifies the kidney, aids weight loss, lower heart rate and treats heart diseases.

CALYPSO

Scientific name: Calypso bulbosa

Family: Orchidaceae

DESCRIPTION

It is 8 to 20 cm long.

FACTS

It is low in calories and fat. It contains potassium, zinc, copper, iron and magnesium.

NATURAL HABITAT

It is native to North America.

USES

It is used to treat cold, fever, sore throat, flu, sinus infection, heart diseases, anemia, cancer, colon, aids weight loss by suppressing appetite.

ALMOND

Scientific name: Prunus dulcis

Family: Rosaceae

DESCRIPTION

It is about 4 to 20 m in height.

FACTS

It is high in protein, fiber, vitamins, fat and magnesium.

NATURAL HABITAT

It is native to Iran.

USES

It lowers cholesterol levels and is used to treat diabetes, obesity and high blood pressure. It regulates blood sugar levels and boosts metabolism.

BAY LEAVES

Scientific name: Laurus nobilis

Family: Laurels

DESCRIPTION

It is about 60 ft tall.

FACTS

It is an aromatic herb. It is rich in vitamin A and C, calcium, iron, magnesium and potassium. It has antioxidant, antibacterial and antiviral properties.

NATURAL HABITAT

It is native to the Mediterranean region

USES

It reduces cholesterol in the body. It prevents kidney stones, acts as insect repellent, improves insulin and glucose metabolism in the body. It helps with hair growth.

CHAMOMILE

Scientific name: Matricaria chamomilla

Family: Asteraceae

DESCRIPTION

It is about 15 to 60 cm tall.

FACTS

It is a medicinal herb.

NATURAL HABITAT

It is native to Southern and Eastern Europe.

USES

It is used to treat anxiety, depression, dandruff, dryness in the scalp, irritation, wounds, eczema, inflammation, cancer, cold, constipation, stress, insomnia, diabetes, kidney and respiratory problems. It flushes harmful toxins and relaxes the muscles. It balances the hormones and regularizes the menstrual cycle.

VIRGINIA SPRING BEAUTY

Scientific name: Claytonia virginica

Family: Montiaceae

DESCRIPTION

It is about 5 to 40 cm tall.

FACTS

It is rich in vitamin A and C.

NATURAL HABITAT

It is native to North America.

USES

It is used to treat eyesight problems, convulsions, skin dryness, sore throat, urinary tract and digestive problems. It boosts the immune system. Women used it as contraceptives.

EPHEDRA

Scientific name: Ephedra Californica

Family: Ephedraceae

DESCRIPTION

The stems are green and photosynthetic.

FACTS

It is a medicinal herb. It contains properties like ephedrine and alkaloids

NATURAL HABITAT

It is native to North America, Southern Europe and Asia.

USES

It is used as an antidepressant and anti-decongestant. It is an energy booster and used to treat depression and anxiety. It is also used to treat stomach aches and digestive problems.

BIGLEAF ASTER

Scientific name: Eurybia macrophylla.

Family: Asteraceae

DESCRIPTION

The flowers appear in the summer. The color varies from white to cream to yellow.

FACTS

It is a medicinal herb.

NATURAL HABITAT

It is native to eastern North America and central Canada.

USES

It is used to treat stomach ache, joint pain, headache and sexually transmitted disease.

ALOE VERA

Scientific name: Asphodelaceae

Family: Liliaceae

DESCRIPTION

It is a stemless plant that is 60 to 100 cm tall. The leaves are thick and it is green in color. It should not be ingested orally because it contains chemicals that cause cancer. Oral ingestion can also cause cramps and diarrhea.

FACT

There are over 500 species.

NATURAL HABITAT

It grows in tropical, semi tropical and arid environments. It is native to the Arabian Peninsula

USES

It soothes skin after minor burns, abrasions, or sunburn it treats skin issues including psoriasis and dandruff and cancer, constipation. It is used as a laxative. It prevents the skin from UV radiation.

ANGELICA

Scientific name: Angelica archangelica

Family: Apiaceae

DESCRIPTION

It grows leaves only, the stem is about 8 ft tall.

FACT

It is an ornamental flower and it is a perennial plant. The root is used for flavoring preparations.

NATURAL HABITAT

It grows in damp soils, especially riverine areas.

USES

It is used for various medical ailments, such as malaria, anemia, fever, heartburn, flatulence, anxiety and arthritis. It is also used for gynecological issues. Improves sex drive and increases urine production. It is used to treat nerve and joint pain when applied directly to the skin. It reduces nicotine withdrawal symptoms when used in aromatherapy.

ARNICA

Scientific name: Arnica montana

Family: Asteraceae

DESCRIPTION

The plant is deeply rooted with an erect stem. The flowers are green or yellow in color. It is about 10 to 15 cm long.

FACT

It is a perennial plant. The plant is medicinal. It should be used topically.

NATURAL HABITAT

It grows well in temperate climates and can survive low temperature and frosts. It is native to arctic regions of Northern Eurasia and America.

USES

It is used to treat sore muscles, sprains, joint pain, insect bites, joint soreness, and swelling from broken bones. It reduces bruising when applied topically after an injury. It is used to eases the treatment of minor burns

ASH TREES

Scientific name: Fraxinus Sp

Family: Oleaceae

DESCRIPTION

It grows up to 30 meters tall. The bark is light grey while the leaves are 4 to 8 lance shaped leaflets.

FACT

It is a medicinal herb. The flowers bloom from April to May. It has anti-inflammatory properties. It should be applied topically.

NATURAL HABITAT

It is native to America.

USES

It cures snake bites. It can be used as a laxative and soothe arthritis. It is used to treat skin sores, itchiness, lices and rheumatism.

ASHWAGANDHA

Scientific name: Withania Somnifera

Family: Solanaceae

DESCRIPTION

It is about 14 to 30 inches tall. The leaves are green and about 10 to 12 cm long. The flowers are small and bell shaped.

FACT

It is a perennial and hardy herb. It has been used for over 3000 years.

NATURAL HABITAT

It is native to India and Nepal.

USES

It is used to treat dementia, arthritis, reduce stress and improve memory. It helps to reduce cortisol levels and anxiety. It increases testosterone level and sperm count.

ASTRAGALUS

Scientific name: Astragalus propinquus

Family: Fabaceae

DESCRIPTION

The flowers are in clusters and it has three types of petals which are: banners, keel and wings.

FACT

It is an herbaceous perennial plant. It grows up to 4ft tall. The flowers are small and yellow in color. It takes up to two years to harvest. It is an ancient Chinese medicinal herb.

NATURAL HABITAT

It is native to China. It grows well in colder regions.

USES

It protects the body from cancer and diabetes. It supports the immune system and prevents colds and infections. It lowers blood sugar level and reduces allergic rhinitis.

BALSAM POPLAR

Scientific name: Populus balsamifera

Family: Salicaceae

DESCRIPTION

It is about 50 ft tall. It can live up to 50 years. It is known for its strong and sweet fragrance.

FACT

It is a medicinal plant that is used as a stimulating expectorant. It inhibited adipogenesis with anti – obesity activity.

NATURAL HABITAT

It is native to North America. It grows well in moist soil and warm weather.

USES

It aids weight loss and prevents diabetes. It is used to treat chest congestion, skin sores, rashes, frostbite, cold and bronchitis.

BARBERRY

Scientific name: Berberis Sp

Family: Berberidaceae

DESCRIPTION

It grows up to 13 ft tall. The leaves are small and the flowers are yellow in color.

FACT

There are over 400 species of barberry and are grown for food and medicine. It has anti – inflammatory properties.

NATURAL HABITAT

It grows well where there is direct sunlight and well-draining soil. It is native to Southern Europe, northwest Africa and western Asia.

USES

It can be used to treat liver disease, diarrhea, constipation, heartburn, acne, eczema, wounds, gallbladder pain, gallstones, urinary tract diseases, diabetes, dental infections and lowers blood sugar levels.

BAY LAUREL

Scientific name: Laurus nobilis

Family: Lauraceae

DESCRIPTION

The tree has dark green oval leaves

FACT

It is known for its strong aroma. It is a medicinal plant. They are edible and used to make soups and stews.

NATURAL HABITAT

It grows well in USDA zone eight under direct sunlight. It can be grown indoors. The soil must be enriched with compost.

USES

It is used to treat wounds, upper respiratory infection, upset stomach, stimulate the immune system, reduce fungal activity, stomach ache, stimulate appetite, eases arthritis aches and fights bacteria.

BEE BALM

Scientific name: Monarda Sp.

Family: Mint

DESCRIPTION

It is about 3 ft tall. Its color ranges from red to pink to white.

FACT

It is a perennial plant. It is a medicinal herb and the leaves are used as spice. It contains properties like antimicrobial, antibacterial, antiviral and antispasmodic.

NATURAL HABITAT

It grows in an area with well-draining soil and full sunlight.

USES

It reduces insomnia. It treats bee stings, sore throats, mouth sores and bug bites, reduces anxiety and stress, relieves upset stomach, gas, and nausea.

BEECH TREE

Scientific name: Fagus Sp.

Family: Fagaceae

DESCRIPTION

The bark is smooth and grey. It is about 80 ft tall. It lives up to 200 to 300 years.

FACT

It is a monoecious plant. The small flowers are unisexual and the female ones borne in pairs. Its fruit is referred to as beechnuts. It has properties like antiviral, antimicrobial, and antibacterial.

NATURAL HABITAT

It grows well in a moist and well-draining location. It is native to Asia, Europe and North America.

USES

It is used to treat tooth aches and congestion. It regulates the digestive system, reduces headaches and mild pain issues when used as a poultice or salve, neutralizes free radicals that might contribute to cancer and boosts kidney function and stimulates urination when used as a decoction.

BELLADONNA

Scientific name: Atropa belladonna

Family: Solanaceae

DESCRIPTION

It is an herbaceous perennial plant. It is about 7ft tall and 7 inches wide. The flowers are dull purple and it is faintly scented. The fruits are called berries.

FACT

It is a perennial plant. The foliage and berries should not be ingested because it is toxic. The toxins are atropine, scopolamine and hyoscyamine which can cause hallucination and delirium.

NATURAL HABITAT

It is native to Europe , western Asia and North Africa. It grows in zones 5 through 9. It grows well in well - drained soil with full sunlight under shade.

USES

It could be used to treat ulcers and can be used as a pain reliever.

BIRCH TREE

Scientific name: Betula Sp.

Family:Betulaceae

DESCRIPTION

It is about 50 to 70 ft tall. The bark is lightly colored.

FACT

It has anti-inflammatory, antimicrobial, antiviral, and antioxidant properties which make them useful medicinal plants. It also contains salicylate. Medicinal mushroom species grow on birch and they are chaga, birch polypore, and tinder polypore.

NATURAL HABITAT

It grows well in colder regions. It is native to North America, however hot, dry climates make it hard for them to grow.

USES

It is a natural pain reliever. It relieves inflammation, arthritis pain, muscle pain and fever. It treats skin disorders like eczema, combat urinary tract infections and cystitis, calms arthritis and gout and fights against cellulite,

BLACK EYED SUSAN

Scientific name: Rudbeckia hirta

Family: Asteraceae

DESCRIPTION

It is 3 inches in diameter.

FACT

It blooms from June to October and it is biennial and perennial.

NATIVE HABITANT

It is native to North America.

USES

It is used to treat snake bites, colds, ear aches, and stimulates the immune system. It is used to treat parasitic worms, increase the flowering of urine and treat minor cuts, sores, scrapes, and swelling from small injuries.

BLACK WALNUT

Scientific name: Juglans Nigra

Family: Juglandaceae

DESCRIPTION

It can live up to 200 years and is intolerant of drought. It stretches up to 100 ft. It has a spicy odor. It is about 100 to 300 ft tall. The bark is grey-black. The buds are pale and hairy. The leaves are about 1 to 2 ft long.

FACT

It can be toxic to nearby plants. It contains properties like antimicrobial, anti-inflammatory, and antioxidant.

NATURAL HABITAT

It is native to central and eastern North America.

USES

It can be used as an iodine supplement and treat intestinal parasites in both humans and animals. It treats food-borne illnesses, such as Listeria, Salmonella, and E. coli. It aids weight loss, kills strains of Candida and other fungal infections but has a mild laxative effect and encourages healthy bile flow.

BLESSED THISTLE

Scientific name: Cnicus benedictus

Family: Asteraceae

DESCRIPTION

The leaves are toothed with spines and yellow flower heads.

FACT

It is a medicinal herb. The leaves can be used fresh or dried.

NATURAL HABITAT

It is native to Mediterranean.

USES

It promotes milk production in nursing mothers. It treats menstrual problems. It increases circulation and treats hormonal imbalance, enhances memory and stimulates appetite and eases digestive problems.

BLUE VERVAIN

Scientific name: Verbena Hastata

Family: Verbenaceae

DESCRIPTION

The herb leaves have double serrate margins. It is hardy and drought resistant.

FACT

It is a wildflower. It has anti – inflammatory properties.

NATURAL HABITAT

It is native to North America and grows on moist meadows, streams and wild areas. It grows well in moist soil and direct sunlight.

USES

It can be used to treat anxiety, depression, menstrual disorders, insomnia, abdominal pains, ulcers, fever, coughs, cramps, cuts and scrapes.

BORAGE

Scientific name: Borago officinalis

Family: Boraginaceae

DESCRIPTION

It is about 2 ft tall. The plant self – seed and grows year after year in an area. The flowers are small and blue in color.

FACT

The seed oil is used to treat degenerative diseases.

NATURAL HABITAT

It is a native to the Middle East.

USES

It is used to treat skin disorders like eczema, rheumatoid, arthritis, swelling, acute respiratory diseases, cough, congestion and fever. It is used to boost breast milk, prevent inflammation, and relieve depression and anxiety.

BURDOCK

Scientific name: Arctium Lappa

Family: Asteraceae

DESCRIPTION

The leaves are dark- green and grow up to 70cm long. It is a food plant to other Lepidoptera.

FACT

It is an herbaceous biennial plant. It is edible and medicinal. It has anti – inflammatory properties.

NATURAL HABITAT

It is native to Eurasia and North America. It adapts to different soil types and light levels.

USES

It promotes blood circulation, improves the skin and cures skin disorders like eczema, psoriasis and acne. It increases urine flow, reduces fevers and is used to treat colds and symptoms associated with colds.

CALENDULA

Scientific name: Calendula officinalis

Family: Asteraceae

DESCRIPTION

It is about 80 cm tall and the leaves are 5 to 17 cm long. The leaves are hairy on both sides.

FACT

It is a medicinal plant. It has antiviral properties. It can be transformed into lotion or salve.

NATURAL HABITAT

It is native to the United States and grows well in warm climates with full sunlight. The soil must be fertile and well drained for it to grow well.

USES

It is used to reduce inflammation and build infection. It is used to treat peptic ulcers, nodes, eczema, dry skin, rashes, control bleeding, treat acne, treat bee stings, and relieve a toothache.

CALIFORNIA POPPY

Scientific name: Eschscholzia californica

Family: Papaveraceae

DESCRIPTION

It is 13 to 152 cm tall. The leaves are divided into round, lobed segments. The flower petals are 2 to 6 cm long and the color ranges from yellow to orange to pink. The petals close at night and open in the morning.

FACT

It is a perennial plant. It is a sedative medicinal plant. It contains natural compounds that have sedative, anxiolytic, and analgesic effects.

NATURAL HABITAT

It grows well in cold regions and requires full sunlight and cannot grow well where there is no adequate nutrient in the soil.

USES

It is used to treat nerve pain, mood disturbances, general aches, childhood bedwetting, and depression. It promotes healthy, restful sleep, calms and supports the entire nervous system, treats sciatica and shingles, toothaches, teething in children, and menstrual cramping.

CAYENNE

Scientific name: Capsicum annuum

Family: C.annuum

DESCRIPTION

It grows about 4 ft tall. The pods are green but it turns red when it matures.

FACT

It promotes vascular and metabolic health. The phytochemicals in the plant creates the spiciness of the pepper which modulates the metabolism.

NATURAL HABITAT

It requires summer heat to grow well. It is native to tropical and subtropical climates.

USES

It is a natural painkiller for achy joints, arthritis and muscle pain. It is used to unclog stuffy noses and sinuses, thinning mucus and letting it drain better. It improves circulation and vascular health and increases digestive fluid production, delivering enzymes to the stomach. It reduces hunger, high blood pressure and relieves pain when used topically

CHICKWEED

Scientific name: Stellaria media

Family: Caryophyllaceae

DESCRIPTION

The stems are up to 40 cm in height. It is hairy. The leaves are oval. The flowers are white and small with five lobed petals. The flowers also form capsules.

FACT

It is an edible weed and has medicinal benefits. It contains vitamins, anti – inflammatory properties, flavonoids and hypoallergenic.

NATURAL HABITANTS

It grows in milder locations.

USES

It eliminates harmful cells and loosen up mucus. It soothes inflamed skin and joints, treats respiratory tract illnesses that involve inflammation, such as bronchitis. It helps to heal wounds and infections. It is used to treat skin problems, such as dermatitis, reducing redness, irritation, and itchiness.

RED CLOVER

Scientific name: Trifolium pratense

Family: Fabaceae

DESCRIPTION

It is a perennial plant. It grows up to 20 to 30 cm tall. The leaves are trifoliate.

FACT

It is grown as a cover crop, forage for grazing, or cultivated hay for feed. It tastes sweet due to the high sugar content. It contains isoflavones, which are phytoestrogens.

NATURAL HABITAT

It grows well either partial shade or full sunlight and you have to wait for 60 days to harvest

USES

It helps with osteoporosis, menopause symptoms, and high cholesterol levels. It supports proper lymphatic function and boosts your immune system, decreases osteoporosis risk, reduces menopausal symptoms, such as hot flashes and night sweats, helps with anxiety and depression and decreases vaginal dryness.

COMFREY

Scientific name: Symphytum officinale

Family: Boraginaceae

DESCRIPTION

It is a hardy plant that is about 0.3 to 0.9 m tall. It has black, turnip – like roads and large leaves. The leaves are hairy.

FACT

It blooms with violet, pink, or yellow flowers. It has been used for over 2,000 words.

NATURAL HABITAT

It is native to western Asia, Europe and North America. It grows well in full sunlight or partial shade in well-draining soil. It adapts well to multiple growing conditions.

USES

It is used to treat pain, inflammation, swelling of muscles and joints, degenerative arthritis, diarrhea, stomach issues, sprains, contusions, and strains.

CORNFLOWER

Scientific name: Centaurea Cyanus

Family: Asteraceae

DESCRIPTION

It grows up to 40 to 90 cm tall. The stems are grey – green. The flowers are blue in color. The leaves are lanceolate and 1 to 4 cm long.

FACT

It is an ornamental plant with blue, white, purple, pink and black petals. It contains compounds like flavonoids, mineral salts, calcium, anthocyanins and aromatic acids. It has anti – inflammatory properties.

NATURAL HABITAT

It is native to North America and Asia.

USES

It is used to treat fever and constipation. It reduces water retention and eases menstrual cramps. It calms anxiety, stress, and depression.

CHAMOMILE

Scientific name: Matricaria recutita and anthemis nobilis.

Family: Asteraceae

DESCRIPTION

It is a hardy low growing perennial plant. It has an apple scent. The stems are hairy and the flowers bloom from May to September.

FACT

There are two kinds of chamomile and they are: roman chamomile and German chamomile. The roman chamomile is about 2 ft tall.

NATURAL HABITAT

It is native to western Europe, India and western Asia. It grows well in cornfields, pastures and roadsides.

USES

It decreases inflammation and calms irritable bowel flare-ups and tummy aches in children. It is used to reduce teething pain in children. It heals gastrointestinal ulcers and soothes skin rashes and irritation.

CRAMP BARK

Scientific name: Viburnum opulus

Family: Moschatel

DESCRIPTION

It is a flowering shrub.

FACT

It contains compounds that enhance health, including antioxidants. It also contains esculetin and viopudial, which are known for being antispasmodic.

NATURAL HABITAT

It is native to the United States. It adapts to most soil types, especially rich, moist and loamy soil.

USES

It is used to treat cramps and spasms. It is used to treat urinary problems and swelling of the uterus.

DAISY

Scientific name: Bellis Sp.

Family: Asteraceae

DESCRIPTION

The flowers are hardy and drought tolerant.

FACT

It has biphasic effects and has anti-inflammatory properties.

NATURAL HABITAT

It grows well in rich and well-draining soil under full sunlight.

USES

It is used to treat coughs, bronchitis, and chest congestion. It reduces inflammation, anxiety and stress. It acts as a drying agent and relieves minor pain and soreness.

DANDELION

Scientific name: Taraxacum officinale

Family: Asteraceae

DESCRIPTION

The leaves are about 50 to 250 mm long. The flower ranges from yellow to orange. It opens at day time and closes at night. It produces single seeded fruit called achenes.

FACT

It is edible and medicinal. It is an herbaceous and perennial plant. It has antiviral and antimicrobial effects.

NATURAL HABITAT

It is native to the Northern Hemisphere.

USES

It is a digestive herb and used to prevent gas and heartburn. It is used to cleanse the kidney. It helps to control blood sugar and type 2 diabetes. It can be used as a diuretic to increase the production of urine. It is used to treat chronic ulcers and fights constipation and helps encourage healthy digestion.

ELECAMPANE

Scientific name: Inula helenium

Family: Asteraceae

DESCRIPTION

It is a perennial herb. It has tall starks, bright yellow flowers and seed heads. It blooms from the summer to the fall.

FACT

It has antimicrobial and antibacterial effects. It was also tested against strains of Staphylococcus, including antibiotic-resistant and sensitive strains.

NATURAL HABITAT

It is native to Eurasia, Spain, Western China and North America.

USES

It was used to treat coughs associated with asthma, bronchitis, and whooping cough. It promotes mucus discharge, aids in treating indigestion and other digestive problems, such as heartburn. It relieves muscle spasms and tensions.

ELDERBERRY.

Scientific name: Sambucus nigra

Family: Adoxacaeae

DESCRIPTION

The leaves are oppositely arranged. Each leaf is 5 to 30 c, long. The color of the flowers ranges from white to cream.

FACT

It is used for wine, juice, jelly and jam.

NATURAL HABITAT

It is native to the United States.

USES

It is used to treat colds, influenza, constipation, and joint pains. Muscle pains, headaches and reduce fever and stress.

FEVERFEW

Scientific name: Tanacetum parthenium

Family:

DESCRIPTION

It is about 24 inches tall. The flowers are small with yellow centers.

FACT

It has analgesic, anti-inflammatory, and antipyretic properties.

NATURAL HABITAT

It is native to Central and South Europe. It grows well in loamy soil.

USES

It is used to treat headaches, fevers, common colds, and arthritis. It regulates menstrual periods and helps with nausea and vomiting.

FOXGLOVE

Scientific name: Digitalis lanata

Family: Plantaginaceae

DESCRIPTION

It is a biennial plant.

FACT

It contains a chemical called cardiac glycosides which is used to treat heart failure. Parts of the plants are poisonous.

NATURAL HABITAT

It grows well in well-draining, rich, loamy soil. It is native to Europe, Northwestern Africa and Western Asia.

USES

It is used to treat heart diseases.

GROUND IVY

Scientific name: Glechoma hederacea

Family: Lamiaceae

DESCRIPTION

The leaves are about 0.79 to 1.18 in diameter and 3 to 6cm long. It spreads by the stolon or seed.

FACT

It is very difficult to eradicate. It is common in grasslands, wooden areas and wasteland.

NATURAL HABITAT

It is native to Europe and North America. It grows along the roadsides, pastures, orchards, and agricultural fields.it grows well in rich and damp soil.

USES

It is used to treat minor wounds, ulcers, arthritis, mild joint pain and other skin conditions. It reduces coughing and bronchitis and eases stomach problems, diarrhea, and constipation

HAWTHORN

Scientific name: Crataegus Sp.

Family: Rosaceae

DESCRIPTION

It is about 30 ft tall.

FACT

It contains medicinal properties.

NATURAL HABITAT

It requires full sunlight and well-draining soil to grow well.

USES

It is used to reduce inflammation linked to type 2 diabetes, asthma, and certain cancers. It treats high blood pressure and digestive issues, including stomach pains and indigestion while also reducing constipation. It decreases anxiety symptoms due to a mild sedative effect

HERB ROBERT

Scientific name: Geranium robertianum

Family: Geraniaceae

DESCRIPTION

The leaves are lacy with five petaled pink flowers.

FACT

It grows wildly if not controlled. It contains antiseptic properties.

NATURAL HABITAT

It is native to Asia, North America and North Africa.

USES

It is used to reduce the swelling of the kidney, bladder, and gallbladder. It can be used to treat headaches, mosquito bite, sinus problems and congestion. It eases discomfort associated with arthritis and sciatica and relieves a sore throat and mouth.

HOREHOUND

Scientific name: Marrubium vulgare

Family: Lumiaceae

DESCRIPTION

It is a grey leaved perennial plant and it is about 10 to 18 inches tall and covered with hairs. The flowers are white.

FACT

It is a medicinal plant.

NATURAL HABITAT

It is native to Europe, Northern Africa and Southwestern and Central Asia. It grows well in full sunlight and well-drained soil.

USES

It relieves constipation, bloating, and gassiness. It is used to treat lung problems such as coughing, whooping cough, asthma, and bronchitis. It reduces menstrual period pain and increases urine production. It is used to treat skin damage, ulcers, and minor wounds.

HORSE CHESTNUT

Scientific name: Aesculus hippocastanum

Family: Sapindaceae

DESCRIPTION

It is a large tree and it is about 128 ft tall with stout branches. The leaves are 5 to 12 inches long.

FACT

The fruits are not edible. It is a medicinal plant.

NATURAL HABITAT

It is native to Spain.

USES

It is used to reduces hemorrhoids, cancer cell growth and the swelling and discomfort of varicose veins

HOLLYHOCK

Scientific name: Alcea rosea

Family: Malvaceae

DESCRIPTION

It is about 9 ft tall. They are annual, biennial and perennial plants.

FACT

It is used to make herbal remedies.

NATURAL HABITAT

It is native to Europe and Asia.

USES

It is used to treat breathing disorders like asthma, helps calm digestive tract problems like constipation or diarrhea and eases skin pain or conditions that cause discomfort, like eczema

HOPHORNBEAM TREE

Scientific name: Ostrya virginiana

Family: Betulaceae

DESCRIPTION

It is about 20 ft tall and lives up to 30 years.

FACT

The wood and the bark are used to make herbal remedies.

NATURAL HABITAT

It is native to North America.

USES

It relaxes and soothes sore muscles. It is used to relieve toothaches. It is also used to treat coughs, colds and rheumatism.

HORSETAIL

Scientific name: Equisetum arvense

Family: Equisetaceae

DESCRIPTION

It is about 10 to 90 cm tall.

FACT

It works as a diuretic and has antioxidant properties.

NATURAL HABITAT

It is native to arctic and temperate regions of the Northern Hemisphere.

USES

It encourages the growth of hair, bone, and nails. It is used to cure mouth, throat problems and viral infections. It treats digestive problems and builds the immune system. It lowers blood pressure, relieves sore throats, and treats burns and wounds.

HYSSOP

Scientific name: Hyssopus officinalis

Family: Lamiaceae

DESCRIPTION

It has flavorful leaves and spikes of blue, pink, or red flowers.

FACT

It is a traditional herbal medicine.

NATURAL HABITAT

It is native to Southern Europe and the Middle east.

USES

It is used to treat coughs, asthma, roundworms, chest congestion, toothaches and nervous disorders. It reduces digestive problems.

JASMINE

Scientific name: Jasminum officinale

Family: Oleaceae

DESCRIPTION

It is about 2.5cm in diameter.

FACT

It is green all year around and is a medicinal plant. It smells sweet and nice.

NATURAL HABITAT

It is native to Eurasia and Oceania. It grows well in warm and tropical climates.

USES

It is used to treat liver disease, liver pain and diarrhea. It reduces risk of heart disease, improves short term memory, mood and decreases stress and anxiety.

JEWELWEED

Scientific name: Impatiens capensis

Family: Balsaminaceae

DESCRIPTION

It is about 3 to 5 ft tall.

FACT

It is an effective treatment against poison ivy dermatitis.

NATURAL HABITAT

It is native to Eastern North America.

USES

It is used to treat mild digestive disorders, promotes healthy blood flow and reduces post-childbirth pain and joint pain, as well as bruises and swelling.

JOE PYE WEED

Scientific name: Eutrochium Sp

Family: Asteraceae

DESCRIPTION

It grows up to 7 ft in height.

FACT

It is an herbaceous, late blooming perennial wildflower.

NATURAL HABITAT

It is native to Eastern and Central North America.

USES

It is used as a diuretic, treating kidney problems, painful urination, and more. It can be used to treat fevers and colds, induces sweating and reduces pain and swelling in rheumatic joints

LADY SLIPPER ORCHIDS

Scientific name: Cypripedium parviflorum

Family: Orchidaceae

DESCRIPTION

The flower is slipper-shaped.

FACT

It is a medicinal herb.

NATURAL HABITAT

It is native to the United States and Vermont.

USES

It reduces muscle spasms, depression and pains, calms anxiety and stress. It is used to treat insomnia and emotional tension and lowers hyperactivity in children

LAVENDER

Scientific name: lavandula angustifolia

Family: Lamiaceae

DESCRIPTION

The flowers are bluish-purple in color.

FACT

It is a perennial plant. It has a strong fragrance, and medicinal properties.

NATURAL HABITAT

It is native to the Mediterranean region.

USES

It is used to treat insomnia, blemishes and inflammation caused by acne. It reduces blood pressure and heart rate, menopausal hot flashes

LEMON

Scientific name: Citrus limon

Family: Rutaceae

DESCRIPTION

It is an ellipsoidal yellow fruit.

FACT

It has medicinal properties. It contains high levels of phenolic compounds, including flavonoids and phenolic acids.

NATURAL HABITAT

It is native to South Asia.

USES

It is used to prevent cancer, kidney stones and increases urine output. It helps your body absorb more iron and prevents anemia. It is used to treat damaged hair and throat infections and relieves respiratory problems and breathing issues.

LEMONGRASS

Scientific name: Cymbopogon flexuosus

Family: Poaceae

DESCRIPTION

It has stiff stems and blade-like leaves.

FACT

It is a tropical herb with a strong citrus flavor. It contains antispasmodic, hypotensive, analgesic, antiseptic, and antibacterial properties.

NATURAL HABITAT

It is native to tropical grasslands.

USES

It is used to reduce anxiety, stress, bloating and stimulates the kidneys to release more urine and spread infections such as thrush which is a fungal infection.

LEMON BALM

Scientific name: Melissa officinalis

Family: Lamiaceae

DESCRIPTION

It is two ft tall and wide.

FACT

It has antimicrobial, antibacterial, and antiviral properties.

NATURAL HABITAT

It is native to South-Central Europe and Central Asia.

USES

It is used to reduce anxiety, abdominal pain and discomfort associated with indigestion. It improves cognitive function and relieves restlessness and sleep disorders such as insomnia.

LICORICE ROOT

Scientific name: Glycyrrhiza Glabra

Family: Fabaceae

DESCRIPTION

It is about 40 inches in height

FACT

It is a medicinal herb.

NATURAL HABITAT

It is native to Asia, North Africa and Southern Europe.

USES

It is used to improve digestion and to treat respiratory issues and sore throat. It eases eczema and resulting symptoms, such as itchiness, redness, inflammation, and scaling.

CHAPTER TWO: TRADITIONAL
USES OF THE PLANTS

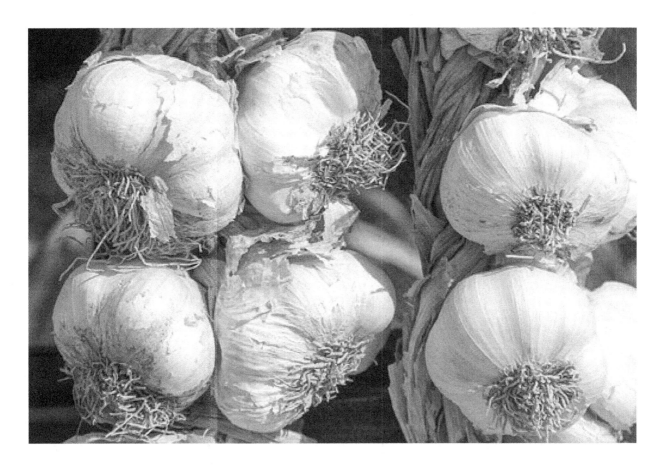

Herbs and plants have been used as natural remedies for centuries. It provides a holistic approach to life, equilibrium of the mind, body, environment, and an emphasis on health. For instance, the World Health Organization estimates that 80% of the world population still relies on medicinal plants; traditional Chinese medicine has been in use for over 3000 years.

Diagnosis and treatment are based on the patient's symptoms. Although there is modern medicine, some people still depend on herbs to treat their ailments. About 90% of Africans depend on and use herbs. Most people still rely on herbs because it is more affordable. People in some countries use herbs as their primary care. It is the most easily accessible health resource.

Herbs are used to prevent, diagnose, and treat physical and mental illnesses. Herbs are used to treat ailments, and it enhances the body. Herbs are mistakenly thought to be safe; however, they may have side effects like allergic reactions, rashes, asthma, headaches, nausea, vomiting, and diarrhea that can range from mild to severe. It can also interact with other medications. Most drugs are produced from herbs.

A single plant can contain substances that stimulate digestion and has anti-inflammatory compounds that reduce swellings and pain, phenolic compounds that can act as an antioxidant and venotonics, antibacterial and antifungal components that act as natural antibiotics, diuretic substances that enhance the elimination of waste products, and harmful toxins, and alkaloids that enhance mood.

People with chronic diseases like asthma, cancer, diabetes, and kidney disease. The factors that are affecting the use of these herbs and plants are gender, age, ethnicity, education, and social class, which are shown to have an association with the prevalence of herbal remedies use.

CHAPTER THREE: NATIVE AMERICAN PLANTS AND THEIR MODERN USES AND DOSAGES

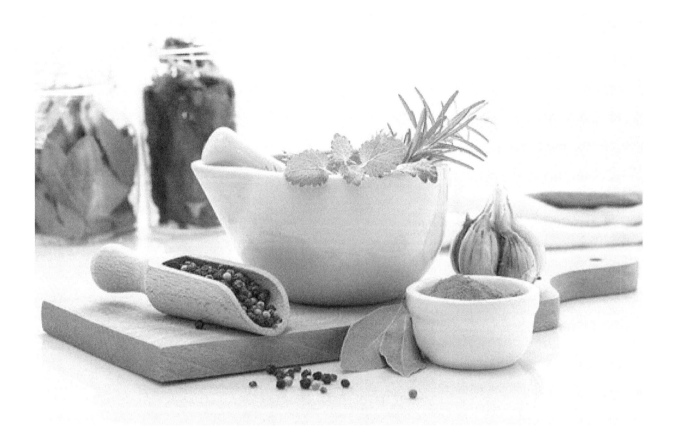

Native American plants are medicinal herbs used to treat different ailments. These plants have been used for hundreds of years and are part of the heritage of the North Americans. Native Americans are known for their medicinal and plant knowledge. They started using plants and herbs for healing after watching animals eat certain plants when they were sick. Their spiritual view is to be healthy, so their health is a major priority to them.

Herbs dosage forms may be administered either orally, by rectal, topical, parenteral, respiratory, nasal, ophthalmic, or optic. Categorization of herbs into dosage forms helps in defining the specific protocols for quality control and stability testing. The herbal medicinal product may be defined as finished, labeled medicinal products that contain as active ingredients aerial or underground parts of plants, or other plant material, or combinations thereof, whether in the crude state or as plant preparations. It may contain excipients. The preparation of herbal drugs varies, and various solvents may be used for their extraction, distillation, expression, fractionation, purification, concentration, or fermentation, which include comminuted or powdered herbal drugs tinctures, extracts, essential oils, expressed juices, and processed exudates.

Herbs can be infused in hot water to make tea. Appropriate processing and dose regulation are required to improve drug efficacy and reduce drug toxicity when dealing with traditional medicines made from herbs and plants.

Herbs have health benefits such as decreasing blood pressure, prevention of cardiovascular diseases or reducing the risk of cancer due to their antioxidant component. They are administered to treat specific ailments. They provide three main kinds of benefits: health benefits to the people who consume them as medicines; financial benefits to people who harvest, process, and distribute them for sale; and society-wide benefits, such as job opportunities, taxation income, and a healthier labor force.

Most plants have phytochemicals, and these phytochemicals are used to make modern drugs. Among anticancer drugs approved in the time frame of about 1940–2002, approximately 54% were derived from medicinal herbs and plants.

CHAPTER FOUR: TRADITIONAL PREPARATIONS FOR THE DARING HERBALIST

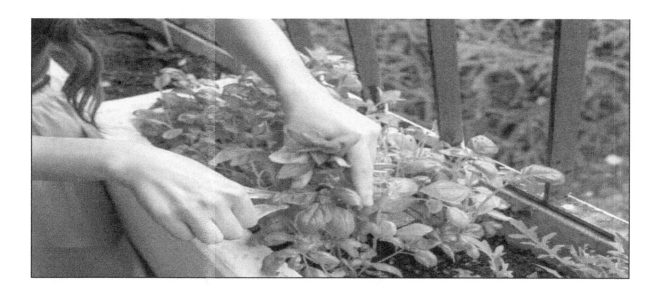

Medications used by herbalists are derived from medicinal herbs and plants. A single herb or plant may contain phytochemical constituents, such as alkaloids, terpenoids, and flavonoids. The majority of plant-originated drugs in clinical medicine today were derived from medicinal herbs and plants. The accessibility of these herbs makes it helpful for new drug research. Herbal preparation has a lot of impact on our health and wellness. It is not safe to mix herbal medicine with modern medicine.

The preparation of herbs for medicinal purposes has been used for over 60,000 years. There are various forms in which herbs can be prepared.

Herbal Teas & Infusions

The most common of them is the liquid consumed as an herbal tea or a plant extract. These teas are the liquid of extracting herbs into hot water; however, they are made in a few different ways. It can be in the form of an infusion; infusions are hot water extracts of herbs or through stealing. Decoctions are boiled extracts, usually of harder substances like roots or bark. Maceration is the cold infusion of plants. This is achieved by chopping and adding plants to cold water and left to stand for 7 to 12 hours.

Tinctures

Another method is tinctures. They are alcoholic extracts of herbs, which are stronger than herbal teas. Tinctures are obtained by combining 100% pure ethanol or mixed with water and then mixed with the herb.

Non-alcoholic tinctures are made with glycerin; however, they might be less absorbed by the body than alcohol-based tinctures.

Liquid & Dry Extracts

Herbal wine and elixirs are alcoholic extracts of herbs, and the ethanol percentage is usually between 12–38%. These extracts include liquid extracts, dry extracts, and nebulization. Liquid extracts are liquids with a lower ethanol percentage than vacuum distilling tinctures make tinctures. Dry extracts are extracts of plant material that are evaporated into a dry mass and can either be refined to a capsule or tablet.

Extracts

The composition of herbal medicine is determined by the method of extraction used. Some are applied to the skin directly. Essential oils extracts are diluted in a carrier oil before applying. However, essential oils can burn the skin if it is applied directly without diluting it with essential oils.

CHAPTER FIVE: HARVESTING PLANTS

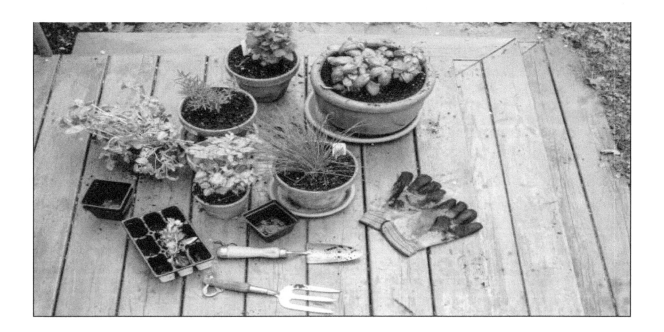

PLANTING AND HARVESTING

Most plants grow best where there is direct sunlight. Plant your herbs where they will receive at least 6 to 8 hours of direct sunlight every day. Annual herbs can be planted alongside vegetables while perennial herbs in the vegetable garden. Plants grow best in soil that is well drained and rich in nutrition. Always water the plants but do not overwater it.

The method used to harvest plants depends on the part of the plant you are planning to harvest. Various tools are used for harvesting and they are: sharp knife, scissors or hand pruners. You can use your hands to pluck leaves and fruits. The leaves should be free of insect damage and other blemishes when harvesting. They are at their peak before flowering. If you are planning on harvesting the entire plant, it should be after the plant's flower buds have opened. If it is an annual plant, cut it off from the soil surface, however if it is perennial, cut off one – third of its stem. Seeds and fruits are to be harvested after they have matured.

WILDCRAFTING

Wildcrafting is the practice of foraging for useful plants from their natural, wild habitat for edible or medicinal purposes. These plants are gathered to be used as food and medicine from their natural habitat. It is for medicinal herbs and is one of the most rewarding things. Collection and preparation of wild plants for use as drugs, special foods or home remedies is one of the ancient professions. Nowadays, wildcrafters gather and dry various botanicals to be shipped to buyers. They search the woods and fields to find varieties of plants, both rare and common. However, certain parts of each plant are valuable such as leaves, bark and stems and they are collected as herbs.

WAYS OF WILDCRAFTING HERBS AND BUYING TIPS

The step thing to do is to know how to identify various plants. A person can start by following a practicing wildcrafter who will put you through when it comes to identification of plants. After identification, the next step is harvesting.

Before you harvest any plants, it is advisable to cut and dry two or three samples of the species you intend to collect and send them to the herb buyer of your choice. Ask the dealer about his thoughts in regards to the plants and ask for verification. Then, estimate how many pounds you can deliver and request the current rate if it's different from the figure on the latest price list because the price of herbs vary from one season to another and it also depend on the company you are dealing with, however if you have a large amount it will be better to go after the best offer.

ETHICAL PRACTICES

- Identify the rare plants and avoid harvesting such plants
- Always pick different spots when harvesting
- Always leave the area in which you harvested from in a better condition
- Adequate caution should be exercised when harvesting
- Be mind of climate change which may affect the plant
- Harvesting techniques should be developed
- Cut the stem or branch at a 45-degree angle about 1/4 inch above the leaf node. For plants with opposite leaves, cut straight across.
- Observe the correct cutting angle and leave distance from the node which will prevent unnecessary damage to the plant.
- Always replant the root crown after harvesting.
- Clean cuts should be made when removing branches
- When cutting larger branches, first make a 1-inch-deep cut under the branch before sawing in the same plane from above.

Lastly, plants either the roots, stem, or leaves , should be rinsed in cold water and dried. Drying of the plant is done after harvesting to give it the best flavor and color.

CHAPTER SIX: THE BEST WAY
TO STORE YOUR PLANTS

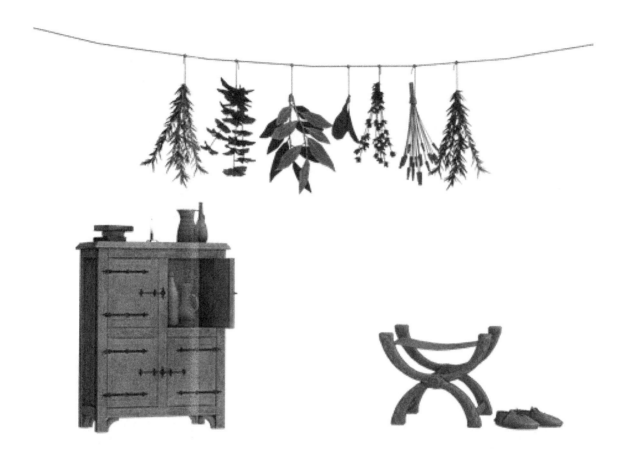

Aplant is made up of different parts with their own specific functions. It is made of three main parts which are: roots, stem and leaves. The root absorbs water and nutrients from the soil. The stem supports the plant above ground level and it's a vessel to transport water and minerals to the leaves. The leaves make use of the sun to make food for the plant and this process is called photosynthesis.

Preserving Plants

The following is the process to preserve plants:

- Purchase or build a plant press.
- Select each plant and tag it in the field and assign it a number.
- The number should be recorded on the tag and in the field journal, together with notes about where it can be found and any other observations that might help with identification of the plant.

- The plant should be brought back to the classroom either in a container or a plastic bag. However, a moist paper towel in the container will prevent the plant from wilting.

Cleaning of the Plant

The loose soil should be brushed off and blot off moisture.

The plant should be arranged on a sheet of newspaper, then placed on the identification tag with its name, a number you have assigned to it, the location where it was collected, when it was collected, and by whom. Make sure the same information is in your journal. Place another piece of newspaper on top of the plant.

Place the pieces of newspaper with the plant inside between two pieces of blotting paper, then between two pieces of corrugated cardboard, to allow air to circulate.

Place the resulting package in the plant press and gently screw it down. As an alternative, you can hold it securely together with straps, or place some heavy objects (books, bricks) on top.

You can dry several plants in the press at one time. Each should be arranged in the same layers as described above.

Check the plants every two or three days, and replace the damp papers with dry ones. It will take from two to four weeks before the plants are completely dry.

Storing Plants

The best way to store plants is by drying it or freezing it while it is fresh. Dried plants can last up to 2 years if they are stored in a dry and cool location. There are methods of drying and they are: oven-drying, microwaving and air-drying. Oven-drying is a method where the water content of the plant is removed, although the essential oils are removed along with the water. Plants are to be placed on a layer of cookie sheet and put in the oven, the oven is set at its lowest temperature.

The plants should be turned over periodically. It is dried when it breaks easily and crisp. Microwaving is the process in which the water content of the plant is removed, however the flavor remains intact. The plants are to be placed on paper towels and microwave for 4 minutes and it should be turned over periodically. It is dried when it breaks easily and crisp. Air-drying is the process of drying plants under the open air. The bundle of the plant should be small, so that there will be adequate air circulation and uniform drying. It should be dried in a well ventilated, dry and dark place and this is to preserve the essential oils of the plant. A paper bag can be placed on the plants to prevent direct sunlight. It should be turned over periodically. It is dried when it breaks easily and is crisp.

CHAPTER SEVEN: HOW TO ADMINISTER HERBS IN DIFFERENT FORMS

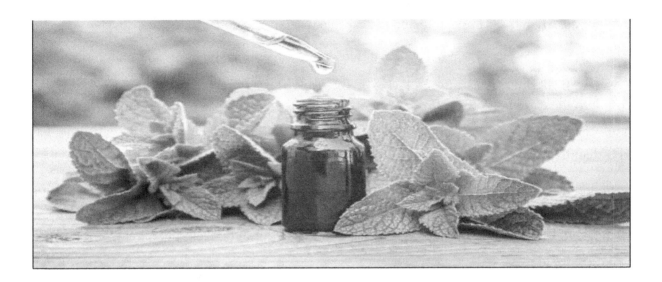

Herbs can be administered in different ways like extracting it in water, alcohol glycerin and oils. Herbs are mostly crushed and dried for convenience and value. Dried herbs can last up to 2 years if stored in a cool and dry environment. The leaves and seeds of plants are used to season food and also treat ailments.

Fresh herbs are grown in gardens or open fields, it should be washed and damaged herbs should be removed before using. Herbal infusion involves the steeping of herbs in either water or oil which can be used to flavor food and drinks.

Herbal Capsules

Herbal capsules are economical and easy to make. The quality and the freshness of the ingredients should be controlled. Empty capsules should be purchased; the empty capsules should either be gelatin or vegetarian capsules. Vegetarian capsules also have their own remedies while gelatin capsules are made from beef gelatin. They are halal, gluten free, free of preservatives, and kosher.

There are various sizes of herbal capsules to choose from, however the standard size '0' holds 500mg while the standard dose is 2 capsules of '0' size. The '00' size holds 50% more herbs and about 750mg than the '0' size. The '1' size holds 400 mg and about 20% less than '0' standard and it is the best option for making herbal capsules for children or persons that have difficulty in swallowing. Empty capsules are sold in bags and it contains about 500 to 1000 capsules. The size of the capsule will determine the size of the encapsulation machine that will be used.

The herbal blend should be prepared in a bowl and the correct amount of the blend should be inserted in the bottom of the capsule at the larger end, this can be time consuming. It is best to use encapsulation machine to get the right amount of the herbal blend in the capsules. There are two types of encapsulation machines and they are: the cap 'M' quik encapsulation and the capsule machine.

The cap 'M' quik encapsulator can make 50 capsules at the same time. The tops and bottoms of the capsule will be separated and the bottoms will be placed in the measured holes, the capsules are placed on top and it will brush into the capsules. When it is full, a tampering gadget will be placed on top to push it down and it will compress the capsules at the same time. The disadvantage of this machine is that each capsule has to be capped by hand.

The capsule machine holds 24 capsules at the same time. The capsules are to be separated into tops and bottoms and placed in the capsule machine trays. Once the capsules are filled, use the tamping tool to press the herbal blend firmly into the capsules. An herbalist or doctor should be consulted to know the right dosage of herbal capsules to use.

Extraction and Processing

Medicinal herbs are extracted and processed before administering it. It starts with the collection of plants, drying and grinding the plants.

Extraction

Extraction is the process of separating plant properties like flavonoids, alkaloids, saponins, steroids, terpenes and glycosides from inert properties. Methods of extraction include the following: infusion, maceration, superficial extraction, decoction and percolation.

Maceration

Maceration is when powdered herbs are placed in a container and menstruum is poured on top and covered completely, the container is closed and kept for at least 3 days. It should be stirred periodically. Once the extraction comes to an end, the micelle is separated from the menstruum by evaporation. This method is suited for thermolabile plant material.

Infusion

Infusion is when the powdered herbs are placed in a clean container and hot or cold water is poured over it. This is suitable for extracting bioactive components of an herb that are soluble. It can be used for fresh herbs to make herbal tea.

Decoction

Decoction is the process where powdered herbs are placed in a container and water is poured on it and stirred. Heat is required to hasten the process of extraction. It is suitable for heat sable and water-soluble herbs.

Percolation

Percolation is the process where a narrow cone shaped glass vessel with an opening at both ends is used and it is referred to as a percolator. The powdered herb is mixed with solvent and it is kept for 4 hours. The mixture is transferred into the percolator and kept for 24 hours. The percolator is opened at the liquid drip slowly and some solvent is added. The extraction takes place making use of gravitational force which pushes the solvent through the herb downwards. It is separated by filtration and the final amount of solvent is added.

Steam Distillation

Essential Oils are extracted from herbs. There are ways of extracting oils from herbs. The first is steam distillation. Steam distillation is used to extract essential oils from herbs for use in natural products and this occurs when the steam vaporizes the plant material's volatile compounds, then goes through a condensation and collection process. A large container is usually made from stainless steel, the herbs are placed inside the container and steam is added to it. The steam is injected by releasing the molecules and turning them to vapor. It will travel to the condensation flask and the vapor cools and turns to liquid. The essential oil will float on the water because oil and water do not mix.

Solvent Extraction

Solvent extraction makes use of solvents to extract the essential oil from the herbs. The herbs are mixed with solvent and it produces a concrete, the concrete is mixed with alcohol and the oil will be released. CO_2 extraction produces more oil than other methods of extraction. Oils produced using maceration are referred to as infused oils. They are created when carrier oils are used as solvents to extract properties from plant material. Water distillation is when herbs are submerged into boiling water and it prevents the extracted oil from overheating.

Macerated oils are also referred to as infused oils. They are created when carrier oils are used as solvents to extract therapeutic properties from plant material. The benefit of macerated oil above distilled oil is that more of a plant's essence is captured in the oil, because it captures heavier, larger plant molecules than the ones captured in the distillation process. This keeps the product closer to retaining more of the plant's valuable offerings.es sleep and treat fungal infections.

Most essential oils have antioxidant properties which free the body from harmful toxins and radicals. The recommended dosage for essential oils depends on the herbs that were used to produce the essential oil. It should be diluted with water or carrier oil before use.

BOOK 3
ENCYCLOPEDIA &
DISPENSARY

CHAPTER ONE: HOW TO USE EACH HERB FOR DIFFERENT AILMENTS

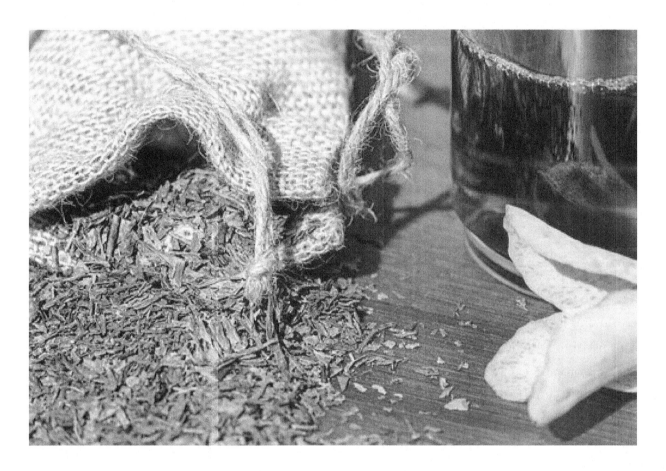

Herbs are different and are used in diverse methods to treat ailments. For instance, the same herbs used to cure malaria may be used to treat colds but in a different method.

There are herbs like peppermint that are used for a lot of things. For instance, applying peppermint on the body topically can be used to treat wounds, diffuse peppermint in a diffuser to create a calmer atmosphere or steam to treat sinus infections.

The different methods used for each herb are important as they can play a role in increasing or reducing the potency of the herbal plant. Thus, if a remedy says to steam, it would be best to steam according to the remedy instead of trying to use the herb in a different method as it could reduce the potency of the medication.

This is not always true though, as sometimes steaming could be as effective as diffusing. In this section we are going to discuss the various herbs that can be used to clear the body of ailment.

1. COLD AND FLU

GINGER

One of the herbs that can be used to cure colds is GINGER. Ginger is a medicinal plant that soothes cough, cold and other respiratory problems. Ginger has been used for years to treat colds and flu. Simply grate ginger and put in water. Boil this for ten minutes and allow it to steep in the water for five extra minutes. Pour into a glass, then add honey, mix and drink.

PEPPERMINT

Another herb that can be used to cure colds is PEPPERMINT. Boil three glasses of water, add five peppermint leaves to the water and allow it to boil for five minutes, then pour into a bowl, put your head over the bowl of water and inhale to clear up the sinus and loosen mucus.

THYME

Another herb that can be used to cure colds is THYME. Thyme herb is effective for cold and flu. Boil two glasses of water for about ten minutes, add thyme leaves and let it boil for five minutes. Allow it steep in the water for five more minutes. Strain the same leaves out, pour the water into a glass, add a dash of lemon and drink. Also, you can steam with some leaves. Simply add thyme leaves to water and boil for five minutes, then pour the content into a bowl and put your face over it, inhale the vapor for about a minute or two this will help to loosen the mucus in the house.

OREGANO

Oregano is perfect for cold, flu and minor fever. It works best when taken internally. The way in which oregano can be used: put water on fire to boil for five minutes, add oregano leaves, then boil for five minutes. Turn off the heat and allow the leaves to steep in the water for ten minutes. Pour the content into a glass and drink. Oregano can also be used for steaming. To steam, pour two glasses of water into a kettle and boil until it is very hot. Add oregano leaves and stems. Boil for about ten minutes. Pour into a bowl and put your face above it to inhale the medicinal vapor. Do this until your sinus is congested.

2. DIGESTIVE SYSTEM

The digestive system could have some kind of element that would stop digestion or cause diseases if not treated on time. Some of the herbs used to treat the digestive system are:

TURMERIC

Turmeric is a potent anti-inflammatory, antibacterial and antibiotic. Turmeric has antioxidant properties which helps a healthy digestion. It helps with inflammation in the stomach and reduces bloating. Turmeric triggers the production of bile. This combats indigestion, bloating and gas. It has been said that taking turmeric for a month reduces stomach pain and diarrhea. Turmeric has antioxidants which flush out toxins in the body.

GINGER

Ginger is known all over the world as a nausea treatment. Ginger is also used to treat stomach upset and digestive problems. Ginger has been used in traditional medicine for thousands of years to cure stomach ailments like bloating, cramps, indigestion, and gas. To take ginger for stomach upset, grate ginger into a cup of boiling water, allow the water to boil for five minutes, turn off the light and let it steep in the water for ten minutes to get all the nutrients of the ginger into the water. Ginger water can be used to curb nausea or prevent and minimize stomach upset. Also, ginger is good for constipation if a person is experiencing problems with constipation, grate ginger to a glass of boiling water and allow it to boil for five minutes, pour the content into a glass and drink the ginger water for at least twenty minutes before eating your meal. This will help in digesting the meal and relaxing the stomach muscles in the intestines for easy passage of poo after digestion. Ginger also helps with bloating, this is because ginger accelerates digestion which makes the stomach empty fast and allows gas to leave the stomach. When gas passes out of the stomach it reduces the size of the stomach and solves the problem of bloating of the stomach. To stop bloating by expelling gas, make ginger tea and add one teaspoon of turmeric, then lie on your back and massage your tummy with honey. Massage until the tummy gets warm and drink the ginger tea in intervals. This will aid in passing gas and reduction of bloating.

SAGE

Sage has so many wonderful benefits. This sage is especially good for the stomach as it helps with digestive problems, gas, bloating, diarrhea, heartburn and stomach pain. Sage has anti-inflammatory and antioxidant properties which soothe the stomach because of its antioxidant properties which flushes out toxins in the human body. It also helps against stomach cancer, stomach flu and other diseases. Sage can be used for stomach problems. To make this sage tea, boil water for about ten minutes and add sage leaves to the water, then allow it to boil for about five minutes. Turn off the heat and allow the leaves to stay in the water for an extra five minutes in order to get all the nutrients into the water. Strain the water into a glass cup and drink. This can be used to treat constipation, bloating, flu and other stomach diseases. It is best to take the sage tea before a meal or as first thing in the morning to flush the system.

LEMON

Lemon when mixed in water has an alkalizing effect in the stomach. Drinking lemon water allows the digestive system to function smoothly because the citric acid in lemon prevents most digestive problems and the ASDA citric acid stimulates the secretion of gastric juices in the stomach.

To make lemon water, cut a lemon into two and squeeze the juice into warm water. Drink this water first thing in the morning to keep you hydrated, boost your immunity, maintain pH levels in the body, kill harmful bacteria in the stomach and detoxify your body. This drink also cleanses the liver, clear upper respiratory tract infections and melts fat in the tummy.

3. EAR INFECTIONS

GARLIC

The first herbal plant that comes to mind when ear infection is mentioned is garlic. This is because garlic has high antibiotic content which heals infections in the ear and other parts of the body like urinary tract, vagina and the stomach.

Garlic has been used to treat ear pains for hundreds of years because it contains Allicin which fights bacteria in the ear. You can either eat raw garlic or mix garlic with olive oil and use it as an ear drop to ease ear pains. To make the ear drop, warm up olive oil, grate two cloves of garlic and put in the oil. Allow it to stay overnight, strain the garlic out and put two drops of the oil in the ears. Do this twice daily until the pain stops.

CALENDULA

You can also use calendula as ear drop to treat ear infections. Calendula contains anti-bacterial, anti-inflammatory, antifungal and antiseptic properties. These properties fight bacteria and heal wounds. Infuse calendula in olive oil overnight and strain. Put two drops of this drop in the ear to treat it.

BASIL

The basil leaves contain properties like eugenol and citronellol which fight infections and inflammations. These compounds are anti-inflammatory in nature so they are used to fight inflammation like ear diseases. As a result of the presence of antibacterial properties, basil is also used to fight bacteria in the body.

Put grounded basil leaves and stems in olive oil for 6 hours. Then strain the basil out. Sterilize ear drop containers and pour this oil in. Use this oil twice daily as ear drop.

4. SKIN

The skin is the largest organ in the body so the skin must always be taken care of. Some chemicals can be detrimental to the skin health which cause diseases like skin cancer and other ailments. So, listed below are some natural plants that can be used on the skin for a healthier skin.

PAPAYA

Papaya is one plant that should be used on the skin for a glowing skin. Papaya has anti-aging properties which means that it is used to fight against aging in the skin. Papaya also encourages production of collagen when used on the skin, the cell is being produced and it makes the skin firmer and healthier. Papaya also lightens the skin, remove blemishes and rejuvenate the skin. It clears blemishes, acne and other dark spot. Papaya also acts as protection from sunburn and other weather conditions on the skin. As a result of the high-water content in it, papaya keeps the skin moisturized and nourished. Papaya is also used to exfoliate because it removes dead cells from the skin and adds beta carotene in the skin which makes the skin's glow and lightens the complexion. Papaya can be applied topically on the face and other parts of the body to remove dark spots. To apply papaya simply blend raw papaya to use it then apply the juice on the skin and leave it for about twenty minutes and wash it off with warm water. Do this once a day to see changes on the skin. If needed for an urgent occasion apply papaya the night before the occasion for about thirty minutes, then wash off. Apply papaya oil on the skin overnight and wash off with clean water in the morning.

TOMATO

Tomato is one of the plants that is very good for the skin as it contains vitamin C. Eating tomato helps in collagen production. Tomato can also be applied directly on the skin to tone the skin and clear the skin. Tomato has a high amount of water and antioxidants so applying it on the skin makes the skin free of toxins, radicals, bacteria, blemishes, acne, dark spots, sunburns and other skin problems that could darken the skin. This is why tomato is seen as a whitening agent for the skin because it allows the skin to get rejuvenated and remove dead cells which gives room for a clearer, smoother and whiter skin.

To achieve the full benefits of tomato on your skin, grate tomato and make a paste, then apply the paste to your skin targeting the areas you want to lighten or clear blemishes from. Allow this paste on your face for about twenty minutes then wash with warm water and wipe with a clean towel. You can also use tomato as a facial scrub by mixing it with brown sugar and using it to scrub the face, this lightens the face as it removes dead cells, tightens pores and firms skin.

CARROT

Carrot has been used for thousands of years as a skin care product even before humans started eating carrot for food. Carrot contains beta carotene which lightens the skin. This also protects the skin from the ultraviolet UV rays from the sun and tightens the skin. Carrots have a high amount of vitamin C and beta-carotene and these two oxidants will work together to prevent blemishes or other skin damages from happening to your skin. Carrots are loaded with vitamin A, so it prevents blemishes and removes harmful toxins from the body when ingested. Carrots can also be applied topically to lighten the skin. Carrots do not just lighten the skin but also replace the skin tissue because of its vitamins and antioxidants content. Carrot juice can be ingested for skin lightening or the oil can be applied topically for the same purpose. Carrot also has anti-aging properties so it prevents the breakdown of cells and aging of the body. To get carrot oil, grate carrots, or blend in a blender and sun dry until the water is totally out, put the carrots in a pot, add olive oil and allow it to cook on low heat for about five hours until the oil changes color to the orange color of carrot, strain the oil out of the carrot and use the oil as part of your skincare product. You can apply this oil topically and keep it overnight for best results. Cold pressed carrot oil can also be gotten from carrot blend. Blend carrots and sun dry in an open place when it is totally dried, put in a container and cover with olive oil and leave it for about three days to infuse the oil. When the oil turns orange, strain the carrot out and use the oil for cooking or topical application.

CUCUMBER

Any skin care regimen that doesn't include cucumber is not complete. From high-end spas to simple treatment at home and cooking, cucumbers play a big part of the skin care regimen as it is highly beneficial to irritated and acne-prone skin. You can simply cut a sliced cucumber into the fridge and place the cold slices around your face for healing of the skin and tightening of pores. You can also make cucumber paste and apply the paste on the face for twenty minutes. Wash off with warm water and wipe your face dry with a clean towel. Cucumber whitens the face and protects it from harsh weather. Also, cucumber soothes the skin, treating blemishes and dark spots. Cucumber has anti-inflammatory properties which removes blemishes and gives a glowing skin.

LEMON

Lemon is highly effective for a skin care regimen. Lemon has antibacterial properties, antioxidants and high pH levels that decreases oil on the skin, reduces inflammation, cures fungal infection, minimizes skin damage and prevents rapid aging. A lot of people can apply lemon directly on the face without problems but some people react to it because of its high acidic content, so lemon could be mixed with other products like honey to be applied on the face or first of all apply on other parts of the body and if you react badly to it then do not apply on your face as lemon can cause irritation on face or broken skin. If you have broken skin on the body please do not apply lemon as it could cause irritation. Do not keep lemon on the skin for too long as it could cause irritation. Apart from this, lemon can whiten the skin in a short period of time. Simply mix lemon with honey and milk, then apply to the face for fifteen minutes, wash off with warm water and keep face clean with a towel. This will give you a glowing skin in a matter of days.

5. SEXUAL PROBLEMS

Sexual problems are one of the leading causes of divorce in every society. From time immemorial humans have always tried to find solutions to their sexual related problems. Throughout these years of research people have discovered some medicinal plants that could be used to heighten libido and solve most sexual issues. Some of those plants will be discussed in this section. The plants are:

YOHIMBE

Yohimbe is a medicinal plant that is used to treat erectile dysfunction and other sexual disorders. Yohimbe blocks receptors that prevent erection. It also promotes the flow of blood to the sexual organs. Yohimbe has to be taken for two to three weeks for noticeable changes to be seen. Yohimbe also triggers the release of testosterone in the male which allows for a higher libido in men that helps in sexual functions.

However, a person has to be careful with this plant because it increases heart beat which can be dangerous for people with hypertension and other heart related problems. That being said, people with underlying health conditions should not take this herb without speaking with their doctor.

MACA

Maca is an herbal plant that is used to boost sexual libido. This plant is believed to be an aphrodisiac because men who use these plants report to have intense pleasure and being able to sustain an erection for a longer period of time. It can also be used to treat low sperm count. Maca root can be added to meals or boiled and taken as tea. Maca generally has little to no side effects on most people but if you notice any reaction to the plant, you should stop using it and speak with your doctor before continuing.

GINKGO

Ginkgo helps in the circulation of blood around the body. Ginkgo is said to be an aphrodisiac because it promotes the circulation of blood to the genitals which allows for an erection. Also, it battles the effect of antidepressants on the sexual performance of men. It is known that some antidepressants lower the sexual libido in some men. Ginkgo herb works to revive the lost libido in men.

PANAX GINSENG

Panax ginseng is also called red ginseng and it is a natural aphrodisiac. This herb also increases erections by relaxing the muscles in the penis and this helps in preventing premature ejaculation. However, ginseng should not be used for more than three months at a time as it may cause side effects. Ginseng can be taken as tea or added to food to boost sexual libido.

6. HYPERTENSION

Hypertension is when the blood pressure, that is, the force of the blood hitting on the arteries is too high. This usually occurs because of obesity, high sodium diet, cholesterol, alcohol, lack of exercise, kidney problems, etc. To lower blood pressure there are some medicinal herbs that could help manage hypertension.

BASIL

One of those herbs is basil. Basil has antioxidants which can lower blood pressure. This antioxidant called eugenol can prevent calcium from entering the heart allowing blood vessels to relax. Another way to take basil for hypertension is by boiling the leaves in water for five minutes. Strain the leaves out of the water and drink the basil first thing in the morning as tea.

BACOPA MONNIERI

Another herb that can help manage hypertension is bacopa monnieri. This plant lowers blood pressure by triggering the release of nitric oxide. This triggers managers anxiety, depression and blood pressure. So, people with hypertension should incorporate these plants into their meals or take them as a drink.

GARLIC

Another herb that could be useful for hypertension is garlic. Garlic has sulphur which will help in the circulation of blood and also in relaxation of muscles and blood vessels. Garlic reduces high blood pressure so it is helpful for those with hypertension.

THYME

Another herb that can be used to treat hypertension is thyme. You can boil this in hot water for five minutes, turn off the heat and allow it to steep in the water for ten more minutes. Take it first thing in the morning to help manage hypertension. This plant has rosmarinic acid which relaxes blood vessels and leads to lower blood temperature.

CINNAMON

Another herb that can be useful for high blood pressure is cinnamon. Cinnamon helps in dilation of the blood vessels which allows for better circulation of blood. Taking cinnamon greatly helps in reduction of blood pressure which would help people with hypertension. You can incorporate cinnamon in your meals or take cinnamon tea with honey for a similar effect.

GINGER

Another plant to consider is Ginger. Ginger has been said to lower high blood pressure and prevent the risk of having high blood pressure because it blocks calcium from entering the heart and dilates blood vessels.

7. EYESIGHT

Eye diseases are those diseases that affect the eye, destroy the optic nerves and impair visions which can even lead to blurred vision, blindness, and in worst case scenarios, death. There are some herbs that can help improve eyesight in humans. These herbs are:

EYEBRIGHT

Eyebright has been used for hundreds of years for diseases of the eyes. It has been used as a tea dietary supplement in salads and as eye-drops. This plant is really beneficial for inflamed swollen and irritated eyes. Eyebright prevents dirt in the eyes. It is also used to prevent cataract and other eye diseases. It can be used to heal eye problems.

CARROTS

Carrot has beta-carotene which the body converts to vitamin A. Carrot reduces the cholesterol level and improves vision. This fruit is excellent for eyes because it contains vitamin A which cleans the surface of the eyes and prevents eye infections. Generally, carrots improve eyesight because the body uses beta carotene to make vitamin A which is essential for the eye.

KALE

Kale is a vegetable that improves eyesight and prevents eye diseases like cataracts and macular degeneration as it contains vitamin A. Kale contains certain properties like lutein that promotes eyesight and improves health. Kale can be made as snacks by baking, boiling or frying. Munch this snack first thing in the morning for improved eyesight or make kale juice and drink it first thing in the morning for two weeks to improve eyesight.

SPINACH

Spinach is rich in vitamin C, A and E. It also contains carotenoids, lutein and zeaxanthin. As a result of spinach's high content of vitamin A, it prevents eye diseases like pink eye, blurred vision and cataracts. Spinach also has antioxidants that prevent or slow the progress of macular degeneration. The results of spinach may not be seen immediately but will be seen over time if one adds spinach to regular diet. One is advised to take one cup of spinach a day to help the retina. It also helps the eye to detect contrast which ensures healthy long-term vision. To add spinach to your diet you can make it in your salad, make a smoothie and drink each day or cook spinach and eat in other meals.

CHAMOMILE

Chamomile is good for eyesight as it prevents sore eyes because of anti-inflammatory properties found in this herb. Chamomile also reduces swelling and redness of the eyes. This herb also contains a component known as tannin. Tannin has anti-inflammatory effects which reduces dark circles, puffiness and other physical diseases of the eyes. It also helps in fighting the skin around the eyes and reduces congestion in the eyes. Chamomile soothes the eyes

BANANA

Banana is good for eyesight because of the presence of carotenoid which is a compound that is converted into vitamin A in the body.

PAPAYA

Papaya has antioxidants which improve vision. Papaya also has antioxidant-rich prevent or slows down macular degeneration. It improves the iris and protects the corneas.

8. OBESITY

Obesity is a health condition that allows the retention of excess fat in the body. Obesity has several other complications like blood hypertension and diabetes. This disease mainly affects the heart so it can lead to stroke or other problems of blood circulation. Some medicinal herbs that can be used to treat obesity are:

GINGER

Ginger has properties that induce weight loss which minimize obesity in the body. Ginger also flushes toxins out of the body and through this method takes out the harmful bacteria and free radicals that could have developed as a result of obesity. Ginger can be used to cure obesity. To achieve this, grate ginger and add to boiling water and let it burn for 5 minutes and then drink it first thing in the morning. Or blend ginger with cucumber, mint or lime and drink as a smoothie before breakfast. You can also blend ginger and add to your drinking water during this the whole day. Within a few weeks you should notice changes in your body size and in your breathing.

CAYENNE PEPPER

Cayenne pepper has certain properties which cause sweating and lead to weight loss. Cayenne pepper also heightens metabolism in the body and this leads to fat being burned for energy. This conversion of fat to energy results in weight loss.

MINT

This allows for weight loss because of its antioxidant properties which flushes out toxins in the body and acts as a diuretic for the kidneys. When combined with ginger and lemon, it leads to weight loss. So, mint is effective for fighting against obesity. Drink lemon and mint infused water to shed weight more easily.

9. WOUNDS

Wounds are breakage on the skin that occurs as a result of surgeries, accidents and other courses. Some are abrasions, lacerations, punctures, avulsions and all the types. The resetting medicinal plant that has sulfur and healing properties to heal wounds. These plants are aloe vera, turmeric, calendula, marshmallow, tea tree oil, goldenrod, yarrow etc.

ALOE VERA

Aloe vera is a rich source of antioxidants and vitamins which helps to protect the skin. The important compounds found in aloe vera have also been shown to neutralize the effects of ultraviolet (UV) radiation, repair the skin from existing UV damage and also help to prevent fine lines and wrinkles.

GOTU KOLA

Gotu kola is believed by the indigenous people that when applied to wounds, it helps to speed up the healing process of the wound. It is also used to reduce the appearance of stretch marks and scars on the body. It is mainly used in making anti-ageing and sun-care products. It helps to keep skin cells tight, and prevents the skin from sagging.

LAVENDER OIL

It promotes the healing of skin tissues. According to a study conducted in 2016, lavender oil demonstrates wound-healing activity and it also shows potential for use as a natural treatment to help repair damaged skin tissues. Lavender oil contains the following component and they are: antiseptic and anti-inflammatory properties, which can help to heal minor burns and bug bites.

10. DEPRESSION AND ANXIETY

Anxiety and depression disorders are the most common and pervasive mental disorders in the United States of America. Depression is a condition in which a person feels discouraged, sad, hopeless, unmotivated, or disinterested in life in general for more than two weeks and such feelings interfere with person daily activities. These ailments are treated with medications and therapies. The following plants are used to treat depression and anxiety:

ASHWAGANDHA

This herb can be classified as an apoptogenic herb which has a long history of use as a treatment for depression and anxiety. Majority of these active components found in ashwagandha have been shown to have anti-stress, anti-inflammatory, and antioxidant properties.

Researchers have assessed the results of five human trials using ashwagandha for stress, depression and anxiety. However, four of the five trials reported decreased measures of depression and anxiety amongst participants who were supplemented with ashwagandha.

Experts have recommended taking 300 milligrams (mg) of ashwagandha per day so as to relieve anxiety and depression. However, it is sacrosanct to talk to a medical practitioner before using ashwagandha.

HOPS (HUMULUS LUPULUS)

Hops are also known as humulus lupulus. They are a commercially grown herb which is commonly used in the production of beer. There are certain components in hops which are sedating and it makes them a useful option for people living with depression and anxiety.

A study that was conducted in 2017 analyzed the effects of extract gotten from hops and the effects the extract has on people with stress, anxiety, and depression. The people who participated in the study were randomized to receive either placebo or hops extract for four weeks. After a two week break, the participants who had initially received the hops extract were switched to placebo, and those who had initially taken placebo now received the hops extract. The study indicated that the hops extract, when compared with the placebo, contributed to a significant decrease in the participants' depression and anxiety scores which makes a good herb for treating depression and anxiety. The study also showed that 200 milligrams (mg) of humulus lupulus should be used per day and this will relieve anxiety and depression in the body.

KAVA

Kava is also known as *Piper methysticum or* called kava kava. It is a very popular anxiolytic herb which originated from the Pacific Islands. There are several types of compounds, both sedating and non-sedating, they contribute greatly to the anti-anxiety properties of this herb.

ST JOHN'S WORT

St John's wort is also known as *Hypericum perforatum. It is* an herb which has been used to treat mood disorders for ages. However, St. John's wort is commonly used as a natural option for depression and anxiety. The usage of St. John's wort supplements can vary from around 600 to 1,800 mg per serving. It is recommended starting at the lowest dose for anxiety relief. It is advisable to talk with a medical practitioner before using this herb. Although, St. John's wort can interfere with other medications, therefore it is important to talk with a medical practitioner before using it.

VALERIAN

This herb is also known as Valeriana officinalis. It has some active components in the Valerian plant which have sedative properties, making this herb a good option for anxiety. It is advisable to take 100 mg of Valerian per day which can help in reducing anxiety by changing the brain's chemistry and the way that it connects to anxiety.

11. BODY PAINS

It is an unpleasant sensation in the body which is triggered by the nervous system. It can occur slowly or suddenly depending on the factor that caused the pain. Body pain can be classified into two, they are: acute body pain and chronic body pain. Acute body pain is as a result of illness or event while chronic body pain persists over time with no real cause. There are herbs that can be used to treat body pains and they are:

ROSEMARY OIL

This is an essential oil which can be used to relieve any kind of pain in the body. It helps in treating headache, muscle pain, bone pain and seizures. It is also used to reduce inflammation and boost memory. Rosemary oil should be mixed with carrier oil before use.

CLOVES

It is a home remedy for body pains. It is also used to treat toothache. It has properties like anti-oxidant, anti-inflammatory, antifungal and antiviral activity.

CAPSAICIN

Capsaicin can be found in chili peppers. It is classified as a natural pain relief. However, the substance can cause a mild burning or tingling sensation when it is applied topically. It reduces the sensitivity of the skin to pain.

FEVERFEW

It is also known as feather-few or bachelor's buttons. It is a medicinal herb that is used to treat fevers, migraine, headaches, arthritis, toothaches and stomach aches. It also reduces inflammation and muscle spasms.

12. HAIR GROWTH

The hair on the scalp grows about ½ inches per month. There are about five million hair follicles on our body. However, as we grow older some hair follicles will stop producing hair. This is when baldness and hair thinning start to happen. The growth of the hair depends on the age, hair type and health conditions. The following are the herbs that can be used to improve hair growth.

GINGKO

It is used to stimulate blood circulation in the body and this encourages new hair growth at the root level. It can be used topically on the hair or can be taken as a supplement. This herb makes the hair grow well because of the combined effects on proliferation and apoptosis of the cells in the hair follicle . It can be regarded as a hair tonic.

ALOE VERA

The gel found in aloe vera plants can restore the pH balance of the scalp and this improves hair growth. It moisturizes and hydrates the hair. The gel can be applied topically. It is used traditionally for hair loss and improves hair growth.

HORSETAIL

This herb is used in making hair products. It improves and strengthens the hair because it contains a component referred to as silica. It is used to treat hair thinning. It can be taken as a supplement because the herb is diuretic.

13. LIVER HEALTH

People all over the world are affected with liver ailments like cirrhosis, non-alcoholic fatty liver disease, alcoholic liver disease, liver failure, hepatitis and liver cancer. Liver diseases have caused about two million deaths worldwide. The causes of liver disease are high blood sugar levels, viruses, cholesterol levels, heavy alcohol intake and so on. These diseases can be treated through medication, immunotherapy, liver transplant and nutritional therapy. However, there are herbs that can be used to treat liver diseases and they are:

MILK THISTLE

It is also known as silymarin. It has been used for years for liver conditions. It contains components like silybin, silychristin and silydianin. It contains liver protective properties. It also helps with liver cell regeneration and reduces inflammation. It can be taken as a supplement. Research has shown that it is more effective than placebo treatments. It enhances the overall quality of life.

GINSENG

Ginseng is a popular herb that originated from Asia and it has anti-inflammatory properties. It is used to protect the body from liver injury, fatigue and inflammation. It can be used as a supplement and it is safe for liver injury. However, it can react to some medications which can lead to disastrous side effects.

LICORICE

It is also known as glycyrrhiza glabra. It is an herb that has many medicinal properties. It contains the following properties: anti-inflammatory and anti-viral components. The main component found in this herb is saponin compound glycyrrhizin and it is used by Chinese and Japanese to treat liver conditions. It can be used as a supplement. It is used for treating liver conditions. This herb protects the body against alcohol related liver damage.

CHAPTER TWO: LIST OF AILMENTS THAT CAN BE CURED WITH HERBAL REMEDIES

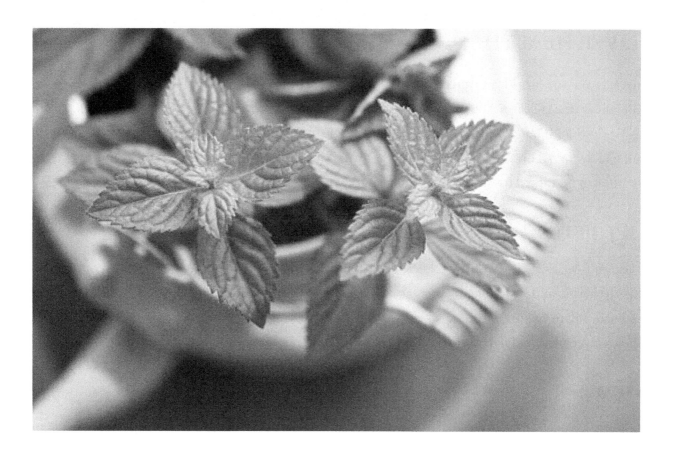

THE COMMON COLD

This can be cured by using the following herbs: peppermint, mint, ginger, garlic, thyme, oregano, elderberry, rosemary, sage, echinacea, tulsi, etc.

SINUS INFECTION

This does not need any actual cure but only symptomatic ones. These symptoms can be treated with peppermint, ginger, garlic, mint, thyme, lemongrass, lime, and lavender.

EAR INFECTION

These are infections that primarily affect the ear. The symptoms of ear infections include itching, pains and general irritation. Herbal remedies that can be used to Battle ear infections are: garlic, onions, apple cider vinegar, calendula, and mullein.

SORE THROAT

This is irritation in the throat that causes pain during speaking, swallowing or breathing. Sometimes this irritation comes with other infections like cold, flu and cough. Sore throat diseases may or may not be as a result of underlying ailments. They could just be due to dry mouth or injury in the throat. Herbal remedies for sore throat include: marshmallow root, apple cider vinegar, honey, licorice root, lemon water, ginger root tea, sage and echinacea.

URINARY TRACT INFECTION

Urinary tract infection is an infection that occurs in the urinary system. These include the kidney, ureters, urethra and bladder. This infection always has symptoms such as: burning sensation when urinating, dark-colored and foul-smelling urine. Fever or cold especially when the infection is in the kidney. To treat urinary tract infection, one can use these herbs: Bear-berry leaf, which has microbial properties that are effective in curing urinary tract infection. Another herb that can be used is garlic. Garlic has antibiotic properties which are used to heal a lot of bacterial infections. garlic can be used effectively for urinary tract infections. Another one is cranberry. This fruit can be taken as tea or juice for urinary tract infections. But caution should be taken with cranberry as long-term use of this fruit may lead to development of kidney stones. Green tea is also effective for urinary tract infections because of its antibacterial properties. Parsley tea is a mild diuretic therefore it can flush infections out of the urinary tract. Another herb to use is chamomile. Chamomile has anti-bacterial and anti-inflammatory properties which helps reduce the growth of bacteria in the urinary tract. Mint is another herb that can be used for urinary tract infections because of its antibacterial properties and its ability to battle bacteria.

SKIN INFECTION

This is an infection of the outer skin which is caused by bacteria, virus, parasite or fungus. This can be acne, pimples, eczema, ringworm, athlete's foot, Lyme disease, cellulitis, warts, herpes, psoriasis, hives, scabies, skin cancer, trauma etc. The herbal plants that can be used as medication for skin infection include: devil's horse whip, onions, garlic, aloe vera, neem, orchid tree, beetroot, red cabbage, merigold, green tea, cannabis, saffron, turmeric carrots, purple cone-flower, eucalyptus, fig, lavender, henna (for impetigo), tomato, olive oil, chamomile, four o'clock flower, bitter gourd, doctor bush, purslane, rosemary, ashoka and thyme.

COUGH

It is a reflex action used to clear the windpipe to allow easier breathing. This reflex happens when the windpipe is blocked or choked by smoke or congested due to infections like cold. Though coughing is good as it clears the windpipe and allows for easier breathing. It can also be damaging when it is allowed to go on for a long period of time. Herbs that can be used to cure coughs are: peppermint, ginger, honey and thyme.

BRONCHITIS

This is an infection in the bronchial tubes. The bronchi tubes carry air to the lungs so this inflammation causes difficulty in breathing. This viral infection can be caused by kissing, sharing cups, touching infected surfaces, sneezing by an infected person etc. This means that bronchitis is highly contagious and millions of people have this yearly. To cure bronchitis most times means to just manage the symptoms during the duration of this ailment till one achieves relief. A lot of people prefer to manage these symptoms with herbs as opposed to taking conventional medication. Some of the herbs you can use to treat bronchitis are: ginger, turmeric, garlic, ginseng, honey, cinnamon, green tea, mulethi, grapes, cranberries etc.

FEVER

It can be simply said to be a rise in the body temperature that is higher than normal. This rise is usually caused by an infection which could be viral infections like cold or upper respiratory tract infections. It could also be bacterial like pneumonia, urinary tract infections or infections of the tonsils. Fever comes together with sweating, shivering, headache, dehydration and general weakness. At times fever could be treated with conventional medicine but in most cases, it can be effectively treated with herbal plants. Some of the herbal plants that can be used to treat fever are lemon balm, catnip (for children), yarrow, white willow, lemon juice, turmeric and honey.

HEADACHE

It is a painful sensation in the head, face, eyes and sometimes neck. A headache can result from medical problems like diseases and stress. It can also be as a result of emotional stress, depression and anxiety, alcohol use or poor posture. Herbs that can be used to cure headaches are rosemary, ginger peppermint, valerian, feverfew, yarrow, betony, mullein, coriander, chamomile, peppermint, lavender, banana, apple cider vinegar etc.

JOINT PAINS

They are often caused by injuries affecting the ligaments or tendons around the joint. There are medicinal herbs for joint pains. These plants are ginger, turmeric, cat's claw, aloe vera, Indian frankincense, boswellia, green tea and thunder god vine

ECZEMA

This is a skin disease that leaves the skin scaly from dried fluids that ooze out of its wounds. Eczema can be cured with aloe vera, cardamom, turmeric, triphala, neem, coconut oil, clove, tea tree oil and chamomile.

DANDRUFF

It is a condition of the scalp that occurs on oily scalps. It is often the effect of irritated, oily skin or infrequent hair washing. A yeast-like fungus (malassezia) causes dandruff. The herbs that can be used to tackle dandruff are: ginger, neem, holy basil, hibiscus, aloe vera, honey, tea tree oil, coconut oil, aloe vera oil etc.

OBESITY

Obesity is a disease that develops as a result of excess fat stored in the human body. This disease can easily be self-diagnosed as it clearly affects the physical body. Obesity often leads to other diseases like hypertension, diabetes etc. Herbs that can be used for Obesity are: coconut oil, lemon, apple cider vinegar, ginger, cucumber, cayenne pepper and mint.

DIABETES

It is a medical condition where the body has high blood sugar due to an inability to produce, or inability to metabolize, sufficient quantities of the hormone insulin. Herbs that can be used for diabetes are: cinnamon, fenugreek, aloe vera, ginger, holy basil, bitter melon, gurmar, panax ginseng and berberine.

HIGH BLOOD PRESSURE

This is where the blood pressure hits more forcefully than normal on the walls of the arteries. High blood pressure can lead to heart attack, stroke or other diseases. Fortunately, high blood pressure can be managed or treated with some herbs. These help are turmeric, lemon, grapefruit, oranges, cucumber, pineapple, green tea and hibiscus tea.

ORAL DISEASE

These are diseases that mostly occur in the mouth. Oral diseases affect the gum, teeth, tongue and throat. These could be cavities, bad breath, gum disease and oral cancer. Herbs that can cure oral diseases are: allium sativum, red thyme, cinnamon bark, lavender, peppermint, eucalyptus, mint, green tea, gotu kola and echinacea. These can be used primarily as mouth wash to get rid of bad breath and other oral diseases. They all contain antibacterial, anti-inflammatory and antimicrobial properties. Also, natural mouthwash is gentle even on sensitive mouths. This is different from chemical based mouthwash. Another reason for using this natural mouthwash is because they are highly effective with little to no side effects. The native Americans used these plants for years to get rid of oral diseases. To have healthier teeth and better gums, use this mouthwash regularly together with brushing and flossing.

STOMACH FLU

This is an infection in the stomach that leads to diarrhea, pains in the stomach, vomiting and fever. It is usually caused by contaminated food or water. This disease can actually last for a few days if not treated but if treated can go after some hours. Stupid flu can be treated buy medicinal herbs. These herbs include: chamomile, lemon balm, slippery elm, green tea, peppermint tea, black tea, liquorice tea, holy basil tea, chamomile tea and ginger tea.

CANCER

Cancer is a disease that is usually caused by abnormal cell growth that spreads to other parts of the body which degenerates the good sales in those parts of the body and can lead to death. Cancer tumors are different from others because of their ability to spread. Cancer can be caused by infections, genetics, radiation, diet and other causes. Herbs that can be used to cure cancer include rosemary. Rosemary is rich in carnosol which prevents the formation of tumors. Another herb that prevents cancer is parsley, turmeric, simple leaf chaste leaf, bandicoot Berry and South African leaf.

COLIC

This is a condition in babies where the baby cries incessantly for no obvious reason. It could be due to digestive problems or the baby trying to adjust two sounds and light outside the womb. Due to the incessant crying the baby could end up swallowing so much air that could lead to gas. Colic affects a lot of babies and can be frustrating to parents. There are some herbs that can be used to treat all cured colic. They are catnip, linden, peppermint, dill, and chamomile.

LIVER DISEASE

These are diseases that occur in the liver. They could be caused by viruses, drugs, genetics and cancer. The viruses are often hepatitis A B and C. Then there are diseases that are caused by drugs, alcohol and poisons. Inherited liver diseases are Wilson disease and hemochromatosis. There are certain herbs that can help cure liver diseases such as ginseng, green tea, turmeric, milk thistle, liquorice, gringo, ginkgo, biloba, garlic, ginger, danshen etc.

LUPUS

Lupus is an autoimmune disease which causes the immune system to attack the organs in the body. The organs that are often affected by lupus are kidney and liver. Lupus has no cure but it can be managed. In fact, the patients can expect to live a normal life span if diagnosed and managed on time. There are herbs that can be used to manage lupus such as: thunder god vine, lotus sweet Annie, green tea etc.

LEUKEMIA

Leukemia is a disease of the blood. It is a cancerous disease that affects the bone marrow which can possibly lead to death if not treated on time. Herbs that can be used to treat leukemia are green tea, garlic, ginger and fruits rich in vitamin C.

PANCREATITIS

This is the inflammation of the pancreas which is caused by gallstones. No, there is no total cure for chronic pancreatitis; it can be managed or prevented if certain herbs are taken on time. These herbs are: emblica which is filled with antioxidants that are helpful for the pancreas. Another one is chamomile that flushes free radicals out of the body. Another herb is turmeric which can be used to prevent inflammation of the pancreas.

ALZHEIMER'S DISEASE

Alzheimer's disease is a disease that attacks the brain cells which causes them to degenerate for many years or lifelong. Alzheimer's disease can erode brain cells and cause memory loss in most people. Herbs that cure Alzheimer's disease are ginkgo biloba, ginseng, salvia officinalis and yerba.

ANXIETY DISORDER

Anxiety disorder is a state of constant fear or apprehension about a lot of things. This could be caused by stress, depression, ongoing worry about personal lives like illnesses and finances. This worry is often excessive and needs treatment to manage. The treatment can be conventional or herbal. The medicinal herbs needed to treat this are: chamomile, valerian, lavender, passionflower, kava kava, ashwagandha etc. They can be taken as tea or diffused in a diffuser.

ASTHMA

This is a disease that occurs in the lungs. Asthma is the tightening or swelling of the airways that prevents free flow of air into the lungs. Asthma is usually triggered by allergens, air pollution, irritants like strong odors from perfumes, frying or cleaning solutions, smoke, strenuous exercise, cold air or other changes in temperature. Asthma may not be cured so these symptoms are often managed to prevent or reduce asthma attacks. There are medicinal herbs that can prevent or manage asthma. These herbs are: ginkgo, mullein, boswellia, dried ivy, butter-bur, black seed and choline.

ECZEMA

Eczema is a skin irritation that occurs in bumps called hives. These irritations are reddish, itchy and also have stings. These hives are filled with fluid that can ooze out due to scratching. Once out, the liquid crusts on the skin and gives the skin a scaly feel. Eczema can be cured with aloe vera, coconut oil, apple cider vinegar, tea tree oil. These herbs contain antibacterial and anti-inflammatory properties which help fight eczema. Honey is another remedy that can be considered for eczema.

BACTERIAL VAGINOSIS

This is a medical condition that affects the vagina. Bacterial vaginosis is when the pH balance in the vagina is irregular which causes itchy discharge. It is a bacterial infection so it can be treated with garlic.

TUMORS

Tumors are abnormal growth of tissues in the body which could be malignant or benign. These tumors are generally not caused by inflammation. And you more do not necessarily mean cancer. But tumors can be dangerous especially when they affect the vital organs in the body like the brain. Herbs that can prevent tumors are garlic, onions, shallots, leeks, scallions, ginger, black pepper, cayenne pepper, oregano and turmeric.

BULIMIA

This is a health condition where a person constantly eats large amounts of food and then tries to get rid of it in order to avoid weight gain. They do this by inducing vomit, abusing diuretics and laxatives, and sometimes working out for hours on end just to burn fat. This is an unhealthy lifestyle that can bring about several negative effects. Most times, bulimia is counterproductive as it causes bloating and makes the person feel the need to lose more weight thereby causing depression and anxiety. Bulimia also causes negative effects on gastrointestinal muscles. This condition can be managed with aloe vera which prevents the bloating and soothes the gastrointestinal muscles, ginseng which helps with nausea, oranges for vitamin c which helps with the damage caused by bulimia, spinach which provides folic acid to ease the depression, and other herbs that help with Omega-3. Omega-3 balances metabolism, mental health and reduces depression.

CHAPTER THREE:
HOME REMEDIES TO CURE AILMENTS

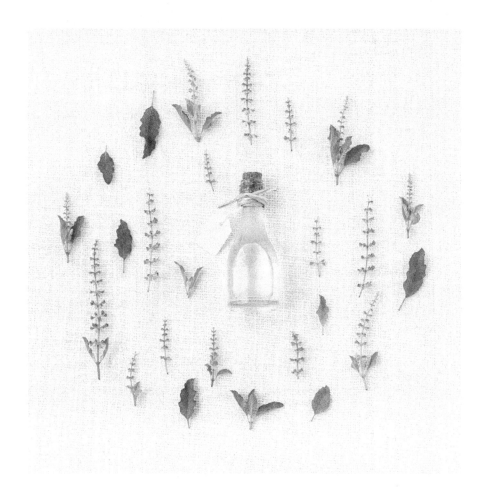

Herbal treatment is a good alternative for modern medicine. These remedies have been used for hundreds of years by our ancestors to treat different kinds of ailments as herbal treatment was basically the only way in which they could prevent or cure all their ailments. Herbal treatment is widely considered a gentle and effective way to treat painful scrapes, itchy rashes, and dry, dull skin.

Herbal tea, capsules, salves and oil can be found at the local health store. The above mentioned are often quick and simple to make at home. These topical remedies do not only nourish the skin, they can also create a gentle seal to protects the skin and retain nutrients.

In this chapter, we will discuss how to make herbal teas, decoctions, salves, oils and capsules at home.

HERBAL TEAS

The use of teas is one of the easiest and most effective methods of preparing herbal medicine. It is an option used to extract the essential properties in herbs. There are various techniques and practices for making an effective tea.

Infusions are usually used for the softer parts of the plant, such as: leaves, flowers and aerial parts of the plant. The herbs that come with softer cell walls can rupture relatively easily and this allows for easy infusion. Also, oil glands containing essential oils and other aromatic constituents are often easily ruptured by boiling water. So infusion is best for soft parts of a plant.

Please note that infusion cannot work for some part of the plants like the root. The best method to use for the roots and other tough parts is the decoction method. Though decoction is generally used for roots,, there is an exception to making use of the decoction method when it comes to some plants. For instance, the marshmallow root is best prepared by cold infusion, owing to the fact that the polysaccharides are easy extracted with cold water alone. Hot water actually breaks down the chemicals of interest, thus making an inferior extraction. Valerian, too, is a root, but the volatile oils are best extracted using a hot water infusion rather than a decoction. In this case, simmering the root can cause loss of the volatile oils that are partially responsible for the sedating qualities of the plant.

The following is the process to follow when making hot herbal tea:

The herbs should be measured. One tablespoon of dried herb per 8oz water.

Heat the water in a pot until it comes to a boil.

The hot water should be poured over the herb and the pot should be covered with the pot lid. Allow the mixture to steep for about twenty minutes to one hour. It should be noted that some herbs should be steeped for a long time to extract more benefits, for instance: plants like nettles, raspberry leaf, oat straw and red clover.

Then the mixture should be strained and drink warm. If it is too strong, the tea can be diluted.

The following is the process to make cold herbal tea:

The herbs should be measured. Fresh or dried herbs can be used. The herbs that are mostly used for cold tea are mucilaginous herbs, bitter herbs and herbs with delicate essential oils. These herbs are: marshmallow root, slippery elm, astragalus, licorice root, peppermint, fresh lemon balm, fresh St. John's wort, and flowers such as rose buds and lavender.

Cold water should be poured over the herb. It should steep for about an hour or overnight before it's taken.

DECOCTIONS

The process of making a decoction is by extracting the properties and components in the herbs using water. Majority of the properties and components found in herbs are water soluble. These properties or components which are water soluble include: carbohydrates, enzymes, mucilage, pectin, saponins, flavonoids and polysaccharides.

The following process should be followed when making a decoction:

The herb should be measured. One to three tablespoons per 8oz of water should be poured over the herbs. Fresh herbs have more water content than dried herbs, therefore, it is advisable to use dried herbs when using this method because it can dilute the decoction and this will lead to the doubling of the amount of herbs when using fresh herbs. However, if the herbs are grinded, crushed, or powdered before decocting it enhances extraction.

The pan should be filled with cold water and bring to a boil.

Allow the mixture to simmer for about twenty minutes.

It should be noted that when making a tea blend that has the woodsy part of the plant and the softer part of a plant:

The woody herbs should be decocted, and then the remaining herbs should be added to the pot, when it is removed from the heat. Allow all the herbs to infuse together for twenty minutes with the lid on.

Allow the infusion to cool, strain the infusion and drink. It can be refrigerated for a week at most.

SALVES

A salve is a medicinal ointment that is often applied to wounds, burns and other forms of injury. It soothes and heals the wound. Salves are mostly a combination of beeswax and oil. There are two major types of salves: lip salves and the herbal salves.

LIP SALVE

There is a simple way to make lip salves and it is achieved by mixing warm olive oil and melted beeswax together.

HERBAL SALVE

The following are the ingredients that are needed when making an herbal salve. They are:

    8 oz. infused herbal oil,
    1 oz. beeswax it can either be grated or pellets,
    a double boiler,

clean glass jars or metal tins and

essential oils.

In order to make a herbal salve, the infusion of the oil with herbs is the first step to follow.

This step allows the incorporation of the properties of the herb into the oil. Oils that are added to salves are essential oils, vitamin E oil, lanolin and glycerin. These essential oils also contribute to the scent, botanical, and aromatherapy properties including vitamin E which is very beneficial for the skin. It also helps to preserve the salve for a long period of time.

The following is the process to follow when making an herbal salve:

Warm oil should be placed in a double boiler. Afterwards, beeswax should be added and stirred until it is completely melted. The consistency of the salve can be tested by dipping a clean spoon into the mixture of the warm oil and beeswax. The mixture should be placed in the freezer for a few minutes. However, if the mixture is too soft, then more beeswax can be added to the mixture.

The warm salve should be poured or placed in a container. The container can either be an old jam jar or small metal tins that work well. The essential oils should be added but it requires just a few drops, then stir the content in the container with a chopstick or other clean implement.

The container should be covered, by placing the lid on top of the container. The container should be stored in a dark and cool place. It can last up to a year if it is placed in a dark and cool place.

OILS

There are two ways of extracting oils from herbs, the cooking method and the non-cooking method. I will start by discussing the first method which is the cooking method.

THE COOKING METHOD OF MAKING AN HERBAL OIL

It is better to make use of dried herbs when using this method. The first thing is to dry the herb and pour oil over the herbs then heat them together for an hour or so over very low heat. Turn off the heat, and let the mixture sit for a couple of days. Finally, strain through cheesecloth.

The following are the ingredients that will be used when making an herbal oil infusion:

- 4 oz. dried herb
- 8 oz. body-safe carrier oil, such as olive oil or almond oil
- quart-sized mason jar
- crock pot or stock pot.

The following process will be followed:

The herbs should be finely chopped or powdered. The finely chopped or powdered herb should be placed in the mason jar. The herbs should be covered with the oil, and it should be stirred gently to evenly distribute the herb throughout the oil.

The mason jar should be covered with the cap and the jar should be placed in a water bath either a crock pot or a stock pot on the stove. When using the stock pot method, the mason jar lid should be placed under the jar with your oil in it, so the glass is not directly on the metal of the pot.

Gently heat the water and oil for three to five days, and try to keep the oil - temperature around 110 degrees. The warm setting on a crock pot is an ideal setting to use.

After three to five days, remove the jar and let the oil cool slightly so it's not too hot to the touch, and then strain the oil through muslin, cheese cloth, or an old and clean t-shirt to remove the dried herbs.

The oil should be stored in an airtight jar in a dark, cool place. It will last for up to a year.

NON-COOKING METHOD OF MAKING HERBAL OIL INFUSION

The heat of the sun is very sacrosanct when making an herbal oil infusion. The following is the process to follow when making use of the non-cooking method.

A glass jar should be filled with herbs.

The glass gar should be covered with oil, leaving about one-inch headroom.

Then, stir the contents in the glass jar together, place a lid on the jar to cover it and place it in the sun (either outdoors or on a windowsill inside, if the weather is cold) for about three to four weeks. The jar should be tipped upside down every day or so during this time that the jar will be placed in the sun.

After three to four weeks when the infusion time is up, the oil should be strained using a cheesecloth. The cheese cloth should be squeezed properly to get all the oil out, and then discard the herbs.

The oil can be used at this point. However, if a person wants to make a stronger infusion, the above-mentioned process can be repeated again. This involves putting the oil back in the jar with fresh herbs and placing it in the sun for another three to four weeks at a time.

There is another method that can be used for making herbal oil infusion without cooking.

The glass jar can be placed in a cool, dark place (rather than the sun) for about six weeks.

The jar should be tipped over once in a while to disperse the herbs through the oil.

When infusion time elapses, the oil should be straining using a cheesecloth and the herbs should be squeezed thoroughly.

So these are the steps by which herbs can be made to get its highest level of potency. Different illnesses demand different kinds of herbs prepared in diverse manners.

CHAPTER FOUR: HOW TO FIND, IDENTIFY, HARVEST AND PLANT EVERY HERB YOU NEED

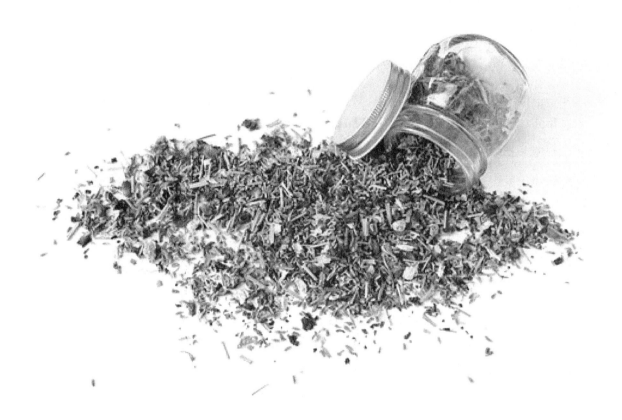

The need for herbal remedies keep increasing globally over the past three decades as almost 80% of the world population rely on herbal remedies either as sole or alternative treatment for diseases. Because of its wide popularity, it is important to be able to identify various part of plants.

The parts of a plant are: leaves, stems, roots, flowers, fruits and seeds. Each organ is an organized group of tissues that works together to perform a specific function. These parts of the plant can be classified into two groups: we have the sexual reproductive and vegetative parts. The vegetative parts are the roots, stems, shoot buds, and leaves, however they are not directly involved in sexual reproduction.

ROOTS

The roots are less visible compared to the other part of the plant. It is essential to know that they have a pronounced effect on the size of a plant and its vigor, the method of propagation, its adaptation to soil types, and the response to cultural practices and irrigation.

The essential functions of a plant are:

- To absorb the nutrients and moisture
- To anchor the plant in the soil
- To support the stem
- To store food for the plant
- To be used for propagation

The best time to harvest roots is in spring or fall rather than when the plant is focused on putting out leafy growth and flowers, however exceptions can be made when necessary.

A garden fork is often used to harvest roots. It loosens the soil around the plant and can be used for digging up the roots. It also depends on the plant and land in which was cultivated, it is advisable to use a sharp spade or hori hori. This is very good for slicing a chunk off of a root crown.

The root can be worked out using a digging stick, hori hori, or cobra-head. Although these instruments require a little extra effort, it works well for roots that travel, like burdock and nettle, or those that are not hard to bring up, like mullein and valerian.

The process to harvest roots is:

1. Remove the roots from the ground,
2. Bang them against the ground or a rock to loosen the root and remove the dirt from the root.
3. The root can be rinsed off with the power-wash setting of the garden hose sprayer or the root can be dunk in cold water and swish around vigorously.
4. However, if some dirt remains, it can be removed with a potato scrubber and cold water.
5. Roots can be used fresh. You can also cut roots into smaller pieces with a hatchet, loppers, clippers, or wood chipper and dehydrate them.
6. It should be stored in a single layer in the oven at 100 to 120°F.

Some factors are very important in development and growth of roots. First, note that roots in water-saturated soil do not grow well and ultimately may die due to lack of oxygen. Roots fare better in loose, well-drained soil than in heavy, poorly drained soil. This is because loose soil allows for easy penetration and growth while a dense, compacted soil layer can restrict or terminate the growth of the root. Container plants do not only have a restricted area for root growth, but also are susceptible to cold damage because the limited amount of soil surrounding their roots may not provide adequate insulation for the root. In addition to growing downward, roots grow laterally and often extend well beyond a plant's drip-line.

Some vegetable plant roots are edible. These plants are: sweet potatoes, carrots, parsnips, salsify, and radishes.

STEMS

The stem supports the buds and the leaves and serves as conduits for carrying water, minerals, and food. The vascular system inside the stem forms a continuous pathway from the root, through the stem, and finally to the leaves. This is the way it transports food and water.

The vascular system consists of xylem, phloem, and vascular cambium. The *xylem* tubes transport water and dissolved minerals, the *phloem*-tubes transport food such as sugars and the *cambium* are a layer of meristematic tissue that separates the xylem and phloem and it continuously produces new xylem and phloem cells. However, this new tissue is responsible for the increase of a stem in girth.

When gardening, the tissues on a grafted scion and root-stock need to line up before any trimming is done. Any careless weed trimming can strip the bark off a tree, which will injure the cambium and it will lead to the death of the tree.

Some portion of the edible cultivated plants, such as asparagus and kohlrabi, have an enlarged, succulent stem. The edible parts of broccoli are composed of the stem tissue, flower buds, and some small leaves. The edible tuber of a potato is a fleshy underground stem and the edible part of a cauliflower actually is proliferated stem tissue.

The following is the process to harvest stems:

1. For herbs with leaves and stems that can branch off from the main stem, harvest the top one-quarter to two-thirds of the plant,
2. Ensure to leave at least a few sets of leaves behind.
3. The plant will grow back if a person trims it just above a leaf node.

Stems are sometimes used for vegetative plant propagation. The sections of above ground stems contain the nodes and the inter nodes and it is an effective way to propagate many ornamental plants. These stem cuttings produce roots and, eventually, new plants. The below-ground stems also are good propagative tissues. It can divide the rhizomes into pieces, remove the small bulb-lets or the cormels from their parent and it also cut the tubers into pieces which contain the eyes and nodes. All of the above-mentioned tissues will produce new plants.

BUDS

A bud is the undeveloped shoot from which leaves or flower parts grow. The buds of temperate-zone trees and shrubs usually develop a protective outer layer of small and leathery scales. Annual plants and herbaceous perennials have naked buds with green and succulent outer leaves.

Cabbage and head lettuce are examples of unusually large terminal buds. In the case of globe artichoke, the fleshy basal portion of the flower bud's bracts is eaten, along with its solid stem.

The following is the process of harvesting buds:

1. When the blossoms are opened, pinch off the newly opened blossoms, including any green sepals or bracts at the base of the flower.
2. The whole flower head is to be left intact but the petals may be removed.
3. Dry the flowers
4. When drying flowers, it should be laid out in a single layer. A dehydrator can be used.
5. Ensure that the middles are dried completely or the flowers will ferment and mold in storage.

The buds of many plants require that the plant be exposed to a certain number of days below the critical temperature before resuming growth in the spring. The period in which the plant is exposed is referred to as 'rest' and varies depending on each plant. A leaf bud is the composition of a short stem with embryonic leaves.

BARK

The bark is the outermost layers of a plant. Plants with bark include trees, woody vines, and shrubs. Bark covers all of the tissues outside the vascular cambium. The bark of a plant can be classified into two and they are: the outer bark and the inner bark.

The medicinal part of bark in a plant is the inner bark, not the outer bark because the outer part is dried out and meant to be protective for the plant. The inner woody pith is medicinal. The inner bark is mostly juicy, green, and has a nice aroma.

The outer bark protects the plant from external effects. It continuously renews from within which helps to keep out moisture in the rain, and prevents the tree from losing moisture when the air is dry. The outer bark also insulates the plant against any form of cold and heat and wards off insects that may attack the plant.

The inner bark is also referred to as the phloem and it is the pipeline through which food is transported to the other parts of the plant. The inner bark only lives for a short time, then it turns to cork and becomes part of the outer bark.

The best time to harvest bark is during the early spring when the sap of the plant is rising but the tree has not leafed out, or in fall when the leaves have begun to change color and drop to the ground.

In summary, the bark of a plant can be harvested anytime in the year but best harvested in spring.

The following is the process to follow when harvesting bark:

1. The bark of a live tree should not be removed directly.
2. The branches of the plant should be pruned off first,
3. Cut the twigs and branches up to approximately 1½ inches in diameter.
4. The outer bark of the plant should be removed from the young branches. The way in which the branch of the plant was pruned will determine the future growth of the shrub or tree. There are two types of

cut that can be used and they are: heading cut and thinning cut. A heading cut should be above a strong node and this will encourage the tree to bush out from that spot. A thinning cut is used when removing the branch to the base of the trunk of the plant junction, or the ground. The whole tree can be cut down or a person can take advantage of a blow-down tree after a storm, however you will need to remove the outer bark from wider branches and the trunk before you start harvesting the bark from smaller branches and twigs.

5. If there are any leaves on the pruned limbs, they should be pulled off,

6. Use a knife or peeler to scrape off the bark and

7. Use clippers to trim up the twigs; this is the content that you will use to make medicine or supplement. More often than not the bark peels off easily, and you can just slice it down to the length that you want or mash it a little between two rocks, then strip it by hand.

If a person decides to tincture bark, then glycerin or honey should be added to the bark because a tree bark is always rich in astringent tannin, which precipitates out, making the tincture gloppy and less potent over time. This is because glycerin helps to stabilize and stall the process.

LEAVES

The main function of leaves is to absorb sunlight and use it to produce plant sugars, this process is called photosynthesis. The surfaces of the leaves are flattened which present a large area for sufficient absorption of sunlight. The blade of the leaf is always the expanded thin structure on either side of the midrib and usually is the largest and most conspicuous part of a leaf.

A leaf is held away from the stem by a stem-like appendage called a petiole and the base of the petiole is attached to the stem at a node. However, petioles vary in length. The node is where a petiole meets a stem, this is called a leaf axil and the axil contains single buds or bud clusters which are referred to as axillary buds. They may either be active or dormant depending on the conditions and they may either develop into stems or leaves.

However, for plants that do not branch or leave. For instance, plants like: chives, parsley, and lemongrass stalks. It is advisable to cut the plant right down to the ground, but for the leaves one-third to two-thirds of the plant untouched. Chives and lemongrass grassy tops can be trimmed from the top. Some leaves are the principal edible part of several horticultural plants, these plants include the following: chives, collards, dandelions, endives, kale, leaf lettuce, mustard, parsley, spinach, Swiss chard, and other plants. The edible part of leeks, onions, and Florence fennel is a cluster of fleshy leaf bases. The petiole is the edible product of celery and rhubarb.

CHAPTER FIVE: HOW TO SOOTHE THE BODY AND MIND WITH HERBS AND WILD PLANTS

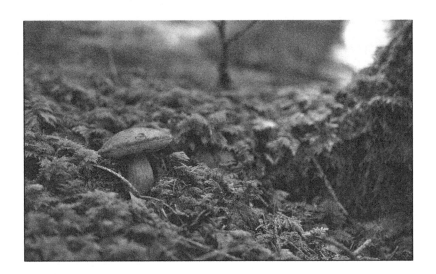

Herbs do not just cure diseases they can also soothe both the mind and the body leading to overall relaxation and reduction in restlessness. This helps induce sleep, cures anxiety and insomnia.

Several herbs are known for calming the mind, improving moods and reducing anxiety; one of them is lavender. Lavender is known to improve mood, reduce anxiety and clear insomnia. Another herb that is known for relaxation of nerves is chamomile. The chemical composition in chamomile affects the central nervous system. Chamomile has a soothing effect that induces restful sleep. To soothe the body with these herbs, when will either have to drink it as tea or diffuse it in a diffuser.

CHAMOMILE: This tea contains soothing properties so when drunk helps relax the body. It can also be added to diffusers to help relax the mind. Chamomile is also used for insomnia and fatigue. It is also used for stress and anxiety as it relaxes the brain. To soothe the body with chamomile, simply boil the leaves in tea. Drink this tea just before bedtime for a good night's rest. The apigenin property in chamomile helps decrease anxiety and induce sleep.

LAVENDER: Lavender reduces anxiety and calms the mind. It also relaxes the body and promotes sleep. It also combats symptoms of depression. To make the most out of lavenders one can take it as tea or add it to a diffuser to inhale the lavender scent for better night rest. You can also stuff lavender into your pillow or apply it on your skin to help calm your body. Lavender oil can be used as massage oil to rest the body and allow for muscle relaxation. Lavender can also be taken as tea to help maintain balance in the body.

HOLY BASIL: Holy basil has an effect on the nervous system which helps in relaxing the body. The plant reduces stress due to its apoptogenic properties which gives the body a balance needed for proper relaxation.

Holy basil enhances metabolism and lowers stress levels in the body. It battles exhaustion, sleep problems, stress, forgetfulness and anxiety. It also has antidepressant and anti-anxiety properties which helps people feel less anxious and more sociable. Holy basil can be added to a diffuser to relax the nerves or taken as tea to calm the body.

PASSIONFLOWER: passionflower plant soothes the body and allows for a relaxing sleep. Passion flower induces sleep so it is considered a mild tranquilizer. It has a cool effect on the body. Drink a cup of passionflower tea just before bedtime in order to get a better night's rest.

CALIFORNIA POPPY: The California poppy plant is essential for relaxation. It is also used to balance the body and maintain general well-being. The California poppy was really used by native Americans as a sedative hypnotic and analgesic. This plant corrects sleep disorders, insomnia and restlessness.

ST JOHN'S WORT: Saint John's wort is a plant that is known for its antidepressant properties. It deals with anxiety, depression and other forms of restlessness. It also brings the body to a state of balance. This plant also soothes the body and mind by promoting relaxation and allowing for free flow of blood.

All in all, these herbs will help manage depression, reduce anxiety and serve as mild tranquilizers for people suffering from insomnia. Some of these herbs will interact with medications so should be taken with caution. Also, it may take a few weeks to stop feeling the effects of these herbs so don't worry if they don't seem to wear off immediately.

The best part is that these herbs have little side effects and are generally safe for most people. If you notice any reaction please discontinue use and speak to a doctor about it.

CHAPTER SIX: HERBS THAT CAN BE USED FOR BABIES IN DIFFERENT STAGES OF THEIR GROWTH

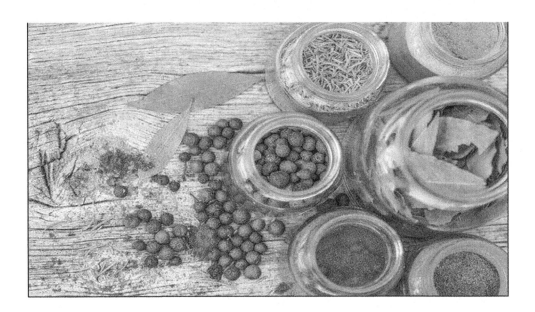

Although herbal remedies are widely recognized and accepted, it is no longer secret that herbs that adults use with little or no side effects may have minor side effects or even fatal ones on babies. One natural remedy that comes to mind is honey. Despite all its goodness, the bacteria in honey can cause toxins which could lead to botulism in the child. Botulism is capable of causing the death of an infant.

When resorting to herbal remedies for your baby, you should only use herbs you made yourself. If you must buy from stores, only buy from vendors you trust as some people mix preservatives and other additives to store sold herbs. These unlisted ingredients can be very harmful to a baby. Endeavor to know exactly what your baby eats. This is very important as babies are fragile hence cannot handle these harmful things like an adult can.

These are herbs that can be given to babies:

1. CHAMOMILE

Chamomile tea can be given to babies as a laxative during constipation to relax their intestinal muscles and help in free passage of poo. So, chamomile helps the digestive and the nervous system. It is also helpful for the immune system as it strengthens the white blood cells to fight against diseases that threaten the body.

2. CUCUMBER

Cucumber has properties that soothe swelling and other irritated skin. Cut cucumber into slices and put in the fridge. When they are chilled, take two slices out and place them on the swollen or irritated area. Let this stay till the cucumber gets warm, and then replace it with another cold one from the fridge. Do this for about 30 minutes or until the swelling goes down. Their soothing properties in the cucumber take away the sting of the insect that caused the swelling.

3. CALENDULA

Calendula is an herbal plant that can be used to treat rashes, eczema and other skin diseases. It is effective for treatment of skin diseases due to its anti-inflammatory properties that heals inflammation. So, this plant can be used for a baby with rashes, wounds and insect bites.

4. ECHINACEA

Echinacea helps to boost the immune system and relieve some common diseases like the common cold fever, headache, flu cough and order diseases. A baby can be given echinacea when he shows the first signs of sickness. This is because apart from boosting the immune system this plant reduces the duration of an illness.

5. CATNIP

Catnip plants have a lot of medicinal properties and these properties help to soothe the nervous system. This means that this plant can calm fussy children. The plant is also good for digestion and for colic infection. To use it for digestion, give a child 2 teaspoons before a meal. For a child's nerves give a few drops of it before bedtime.

6. LICORICE

Licorice is a plant that is used to treat upper respiratory tract problems like the common cold, fever, sore throat, sinus infections and inflammation in the digestive system. You can give a child licorice candy to lick or give them licorice tea or syrup to drink for cold and flu.

7. BELLADONNA

Belladonna is used for a lot of childhood diseases like measles, headache, difficulty in falling asleep, fever and swollen glands. Belladonna is often used when the child has fever and other symptoms as a result of fever.

8. FENNEL

Fennel is an herbal medicine used to treat bloating, loss of appetite, heartburn, gas, digestive problems and colic in infants. Fennel herb is also used to treat cough, bronchitis, sinus infection, cold and flu. It can also be used to treat bed-wetting and visual problems. So, fennel herb is fine for children with digestive problems, constipation and upper respiratory tract issues. This herb could be more preferable than over-the-counter medication as this may have lesser side effects than chemically manufactured medication. You can give fennel herb to children in tea just before a meal to aid in digestion or other conditions.

9. MINT

Mint is good for babies as it reduces or treats stomach flu and other stomach problems like indigestion, nausea and cramps. Mint also helps the baby with flu too. A baby can start eating mints once they start eating solids. This is usually around six months of age.

10. TURMERIC

Adding turmeric to meals can make a baby's system development better as turmeric boosts the immune system. Add a dash of turmeric to meals regularly for best results.

BOOK 4
MOST COMMON HOMEMADE REMEDIES

INTRODUCTION

For years, even before the colonists settled in America, the native Americans had used different plants as medicine to treat various ailments. These plants have continued to play an essential role in the production of medicine by pharmaceuticals all over the world.

The native Americans noticed that sick animals would eat certain plants and got cured. With the knowledge obtained from observing these animals, they took note of some plants, replanted, and used them for medicinal purposes. We will discuss how to use some of these herbs for the prevention and management of diseases in this book.

No matter how effective chemical-based medications are, they are still considered to be necessary evil by a lot of people because, unlike natural remedies, most manufactured medications have side effects due to the chemical processes they are exposed to in the course of production. In addition, chemicals are often added to medication either as preservatives or enhancers.

Before the advancement of science and the widespread use of chemicals in medicine manufacturing, people used homemade remedies to effectively prevent, manage and cure various diseases. These remedies that seemed to have been ignored at the advent of science are still quite effective and can be used to treat many conditions ranging from the common cold to more serious ailments.

In recent years, people are more conscious of what they put into their bodies — and their fears are justified seeing all the side effects some medications have had on their users and how many medications have had to be pulled out of the market by the FDA — so, many people try to know exactly what their medication is made of and the chemicals they contain.

People also try to go as natural as possible in their treatments, as most natural remedies do not have extreme side effects. The need to control what they accept as treatment has led people to research the herbs used to treat ailments in traditional medicine to see if they were of any use and check if they are a healthier option than the chemical additives and preservatives over-the-counter medication and supplements they use.

Research has shown that many herbs which were resorted to actually contain properties that make them efficient to battle the diseases they were used to treat. This has made a lot of people return to adding medicinal herbs to their diet to prevent and manage certain health conditions. Most of these herbs are cheap, have minimal or no side effects, and are readily available as they can be found in the average American kitchen or garden.

CHAPTER ONE: SAGE REMEDIES

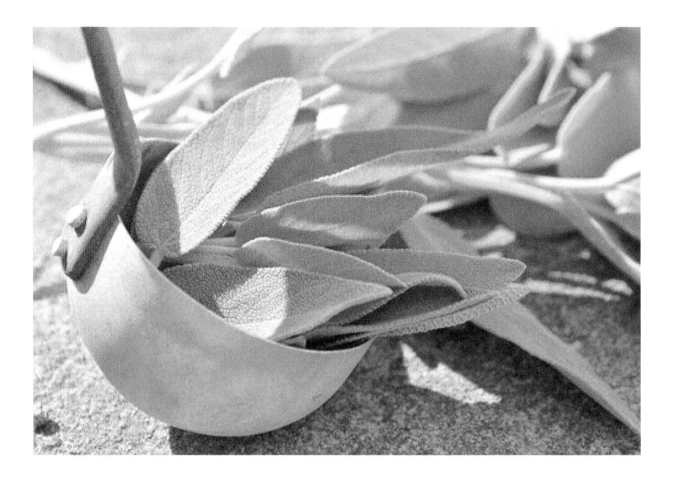

Sage is a medicinal plant that has been used for years by the native Americans to heal various ailments. Today sage is still used for treatment of diseases. Some of the ways you can consume this medicinal herb is by making it a regular part of your diet. You can do so by putting it in soup, making butter with it, adding it in tomato sauce or serving it together with an omelet.

This herb is very beneficial as it cures headache, sore throat, reduces oxidative stress in the body using its antioxidants. Sage protects against bacterial and viral infections due to its antibacterial, antiviral and anti-inflammatory properties. Sage also helps with digestive tract problems. In addition, sage has been found to promote good mood, reduce depression and anxiety. Sage also protects the brain against memory loss which helps people suffering from Alzheimer's disease.

Sage is beneficial to the skin as it kills bacteria. Burning sage helps to release negative ions which improves moods in people. Furthermore, sage boosts energy levels as it releases positive energy. Sage helps reduce excessive sweating. It is rich in magnesium and vitamin C and these properties slow down the sweat glands. Also, sage leaves contain tannic acid which restricts the sweat glands therefore reducing perspiration.

SAGE AS DEODORANT

It is also worthy of note that sage can effectively minimize body odor due to the fact that it reduces the bacteria that produces this odor. Sage does not just cover the bad smell but it stops the smell altogether.

Below are the steps to follow in order to make sage natural deodorant.

To prepare this deodorant you will need:

- a measuring cup.
- Empty deodorant containers
- A storage jar.

You also need these ingredients:

- 1/3 cup sage leaves
- 1/4 cup coconut oil
- 1/3 cup dried lavender
- 1/3 cup of almond oil.
- Half cup infused herbal oil
- 20 drops of sage
- 2 tablespoon baking soda
- 2 ounces beeswax

This is the method of preparation:

Add melted coconut oil in a jar then at almond oil and pour in the herbs. Mix these together and place the jar in a dark corner of the room for about four weeks in order to have the herbs properly infused in oil. After four weeks, strain the herbs out and pour the oil into a heavy based pot. Pour the beeswax into another heavy based pot and place these two pots over low heat on a double burner. Once the beeswax melts, turn off the heat and pour the essential oil into the melted beeswax. Then pour in the baking soda. Stir properly for minutes till the mixture thickens slightly. Pour the mixture into the empty deodorant containers. Let it set for a few hours before use.

- SAGE FOR COUGH

Sage is highly effective for cough, cold and sinus congestion. Some people even swear that sage is better than some cough medicines they have taken. Here is a simple homemade remedy to treat cough without resorting to over-the-counter medication.

You will need the following ingredients:

- One cup of fresh sage leaves
- 1 cup of honey
- A Mason jar with a seal

Preparation:

- Wash and dry the sage leaves
- Pour the leaves into the mason jar.
- Pour honey over the sage leaves.
- Stir the mixture and let it sit for about ten days.
- Take two tablespoons morning and evening for cough.
- When it is finished, use the sage leaves to make tea.

SAGE TEA FOR COLDs

You will need for this recipe:

- About 40 fresh sage leaves.
- 4 cups water
- 2 tablespoon ginger
- 2 tablespoons honey

Preparation:

- Pour the sage into a kettle, add water and boil.
- Let it simmer for about 10 minutes then turn off the heat.
- Strain the water.
- Add ginger and honey.
- Serve hot.

CHAPTER TWO: BLACKBERRY REMEDIES

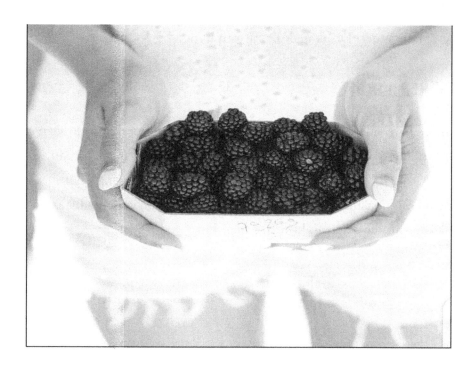

Blackberry is popularly known as a medicinal plant. The leaves, roots and berries are used in the production of medicine. Blackberry can be used as treatment for diarrhea, diabetes, inflammation, prevention of cancer, oral diseases and throat irritation.

Blackberry had been used by their Native Americans for years to cure numerous ailments including toothache, sore throat, mouth ulcer, hemorrhoids, minor bleeding, dysentery, whooping cough and diarrhea.

The natives mainly used Blackberry leaf tea for sore throat and mouth ulcers. It has now been discovered that the leaves contain vitamin C, hydrolysable tannins and flavonoids. These compounds are the reason behind blackberry's effectiveness in treating diarrhea and other stomach infections. Blackberry extract has always been used in traditional medicine and has been proven to help in production of collagen and elastin which gives the human body elasticity flexibility and suppleness. Therefore, Blackberry is quite beneficial to the skin.

The vitamins, antioxidants and minerals in blackberries provide a host of health benefits for humans. The antioxidant, anti-inflammatory and anti-microbial properties combat diabetes and different kinds of cancer. The antioxidants also fight against the negative impact of free radicals which causes aging and some diseases in the body. Blackberries being low in potassium, sodium and phosphorus are seen to be kidney friendly as they prevent the formation of kidney stones.

Below are some blackberry natural remedies for prevention, management and cure of diseases.

BLACKBERRY TEA

Blackberry leaves contain vitamins, flavonoids and hydrolysable tannins which makes it the perfect medication for inflammation in the digestive system.

Boil the leaves and strain the water. Drink it alone or with honey.

BLACKBERRY SEED OIL

Blackberry seed oil helps fight skin conditions like eczema and irritation thanks to its high vitamin C content. Vitamin C helps fight wrinkles, acne and other skin diseases. Blackberry seed oil can also moisturize the hair and scalp. It helps grow silky hair and treats split ends. Blackberries, being high in antioxidants, fight free radicals. This makes it an essential ingredient in most facial masks. You can mix blackberry oil with honey and milk. Apply this mask on your face daily to have glowing skin.

CHAPTER THREE: WILLOW REMEDIES

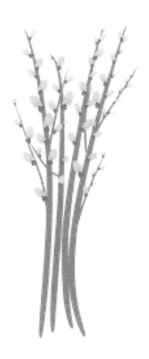

Willow is a native shrub in the northern hemisphere. This plant has a lot of medicinal benefits. The willow is used for several things and one of them is production of medicine.

The native Americans used willow as a pain reliever, diarrhea, even skin tone, joint pain, headache, gout, arthritis and many other uses. It was later discovered the willow contained acetylsalicylic acid which is a pain reliever. Willow's ingredient salicin is used in aspirin production as it is a pain reliever. Some people even prefer using willow bark to using aspirin or other pain relievers because of its naturalness.

Willow leaves are also used to treat fever, skin problems and oral diseases. The bark of the Willow soothes irritated skin, alleviates acne and closes pores as it is anti-inflammatory and anti-bacterial. Willow bark tea is useful for people with swelling and joint pains. It is also used to alleviate the common cold and fever. Willow bark has exfoliating properties as well so it exfoliates the skin and scalp. Because of its pain-relieving properties, willow is sometimes termed nature's aspirin. Once the salicin in willow enters into the bloodstream it relieves pain and reduces inflammation. It is said that willow has a lesser side effect on the human body than aspirin and Ibuprofen. This is the reason why some people prefer taking willow bark tea for pain instead.

Willow is an important part of acne medication as its salicin content has been used to produce a lot of acne medication. So, it follows that willow can be used to effectively clear acne, black spots, and other skin blemishes. In view of the fact that willow contains beta hydroxy acid which is an exfoliating property that reduces signs of aging on the human body, willow can be effectively used to remove fine lines, wrinkles and to firm the body.

People have used willow for saggy breasts, stretch marks and other signs of weak elasticity on the body. So, it is safe to say that willow helps preserve youthfulness and firmer skin.

WILLOW BARK TEA

- Add 2 tablespoons of willow bark to 4 glasses of water and boil for 10 minutes.
- Turn off the heat and allow it to steep in the water for about 40 minutes.
- Strain out the water.
- Add honey to this drink.

Drink four cups to get relief from pains.

CHAPTER FOUR: CEDAR REMEDIES

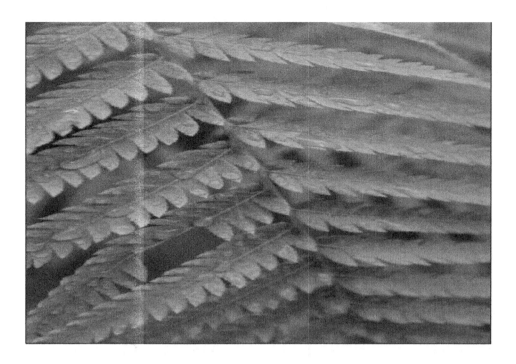

Native Americans consider cedar to be sacred and even used it in their spiritual ceremonies. Apart from these ceremonial uses, cedar has a lot of medicinal benefits. Cedar can be used to fight rheumatism, joint pains, digestive tract issues and fungal infections. If you drink cedar, you will notice a reduction in fever, common cold and even flu. Cedar being a medicinal plant contains vitamin C in large numbers. Cedar has healing properties so it can be used to minimize cough and even bronchitis. Cedar also combats antiviral properties that is why cedar oil is used for antiviral, antifungal and anti-inflammatory diseases.

In addition to all these benefits, cedar has a good smell so it can be used for aromatic therapy. To get the highest benefits from this oil, put it in your diffuser, bath water, shower gel or mix it with jojoba oil and apply it on the skin. The smell of cedar comes from its compound thujaplicin.

The smell of cedar actively repels insects. Put cedar oil in your diffuser or in a spray can and spray it in your home to repel the bugs.

CEDAR TEA

To make this tea:

- Add 2 cups of soda in 4 cups of boiling water.

- Allow it to bowl for 10 minutes until the water changes color to golden brown.
- Strain disorder and add honey to the water.
- Serve hot.

CEDAR OIL STEAM

- Add 3 drops of cedar oil and a tablespoon of cedar bark to water and allow it to soak for 10 minutes.
- Put the kettle on the stove and let it boil for 10 minutes.
- Turn off the heat and let the cedar bark steep for about 5 minutes.
- Pour the water into a bowl.
- Put your face over it and cover your hair with a towel.
- Inhale this steam for 15 minutes.

This steam is effective for flu, the common cold and sinus congestion.

CEDAR OIL DIFFUSER

Cedar oil fragrance repels insects and freshens the atmosphere in a room. Simply add four drops of this essential oil into your diffuser and let it stay overnight. This will repel insects and clear your respiratory tract. The native Americans use cedar to purify the home. This was done by burning cedar to release positive energies and clear the atmosphere of negative energies. Burning cedar can actually clear your mind, freshen the air in your room and also energize you.

MOST COMMON HOMEMADE REMEDIES

CHAPTER FIVE: HONEY REMEDIES

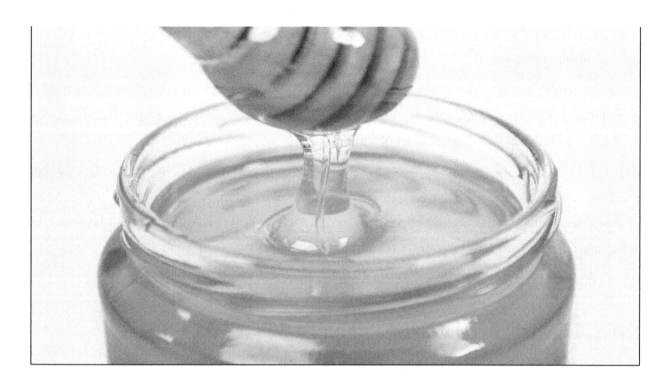

Native Americans collected honey by using smoke to distract the bees before taking the honeycomb. The indigenous people obtained their honey from the bee *melipona beecheii. Prior to that,* humans have used honey for about 8000 years in traditional medicine. Honey was the most important drug in ancient Egyptian medicine as it was an essential ingredient in about 500 different medications from headache to embalmment. Even modern science uses honey in various medications and supplements.

Natural honey contains about 200 substances which includes amino acids, vitamins, minerals and enzymes and can be taken on its own orally, or applied as ointment. Honey is universally recognized for its antioxidants, antibacterial and antifungal properties. It is widely used to heal wounds, boost immunity, digestion, general gut health and sore throat. The antioxidants compound in honey which is known as polyphenols act as prevention to cell damage, slows the aging process and prevents heart diseases in humans. The antioxidants in honey have been found to reduce the risk of heart attacks, strokes and even some types of cancer.

Honey dilate the arteries that lead to the heart thereby allowing the free flow of blood to the heart. This dilation also helps prevent blood clotting in these arteries which in turn prevents heart attacks and strokes. When honey is taken as an alternative for sugar, it can bring down bad cholesterol levels in noticeable amounts.

Honey is also used for stings such as bee stings. Honey itself is balmy in nature and it has soothing properties so it can be applied on the strings as soothing balm. This minimizes itching and helps maintain the affected skin.

Honey has rejuvenating properties so it effectively heals cracked skin, wounds and other skin diseases like eczema, dandruff etc. Applying honey to the area surgery sites prevents post-surgery infections. People who apply honey to their surgery sites daily find out it reduces scar formation, heals wounds faster and overall leaves them with beautiful, healthy skin. This skin regeneration comes as a result of the bioactive compounds present in honey. Also, honey contains hydrogen peroxide which is an antiseptic. This antiseptic prevents the wound from getting infested with germs.

Honey prevents cell damage, aids in the production of collagen and slows the aging process. It has been discovered that applying honey and milk mixture on the face for minutes every night helps maintain a youthful look as it helps with wrinkles and other signs of aging.

Honey is also perfect for sore throats, the common cold and cough. Honey is a preferable, natural and cheaper treatment for some ailments associated with the upper respiratory tract infection. It is more preferred as it is readily available, cheap and has no side effects. Honey also acts as a cough suppressant. It's little wonder that honey has played an essential part in our food and medicine for thousands of years.

These are common remedies for honey you can make in the comfort of your home.

HONEY, LEMON AND GINGER FOR COLD AND COUGH

Ginger is rich in anti-inflammatory properties and also good for immune system boost. Blend honey, lemon and ginger together. Then boil water and add the honey-lemon-ginger mixture to the boiling water for a few minutes. Take it down, strain and drink this twice daily for fast results.

HONEY AND GINGER FOR SORE THROATS

Grate ginger and add to boiling water. Let it boil for a few minutes then take it down, add two tablespoons of honey and drink. Gargle the water at intervals for better results. You can also mix two tablespoons of honey with a warm glass of water or tea, and drink as required.

CINNAMON AND HONEY FOR HYPERTENSION

Mix half a teaspoon of cinnamon powder and one teaspoon honey in half glass water and drink it. Eating cinnamon helps in reducing systolic blood pressure.

HONEY AND SUGAR FOR CRACKED HEELS

The antibacterial properties in honey and the exfoliating properties in sugar work together to repair cracked heels. Mix these two ingredients together and apply on the cracked part of the heels. Let it sit for about fifteen minutes then wash it off. Apply honey there as normal lotion till the cracks heal.

HONEY AND SUGAR FOR FACIAL SCRUB

Mix brown sugar with honey for an exfoliating scrub. This scrub removes dead cells, heals cracked lips and rejuvenates the skin.

HONEY FOR INSOMNIA

Honey helps to induce melatonin, the hormone your body uses to restore itself during sleep. Melatonin is a hormone released at night, which guides the body in its sleep–wake cycle. Sometimes melatonin is prescribed by doctors as a dietary supplement to treat cases of short-term insomnia. When you drink honey at night, its sugars heighten the insulin levels, which in turn releases tryptophan. The tryptophan becomes serotonin, and finally becomes melatonin. This is the process through which raw honey helps with insomnia. Add a tablespoon to warm milk to increase melatonin and induce sleep instead of resorting to sleeping tablets or staying awake all night.

CINNAMON AND HONEY FOR SKIN DISEASES

Honey eliminates dead skin cells while cinnamon fades acne scars, blemishes and dark spots. Together these two regenerate the skin. Warm three tablespoons of honey, then add a tablespoon of cinnamon to make a paste. Apply this paste to the face and let it sit for ten minutes. Thereafter, wash it off and dab it with a clean face towel. Do this twice daily till skin regains its flawless, youthful look.

HONEY AND CINNAMON DRINK

Being antioxidants, honey and cinnamon are a powerful combination for treating a lot of ailments apart from skin issues. You can make honey and cinnamon drinks as a pre-workout drink. This drink helps keep one energized during workout sessions and aids in fat burn as well. Also, one cup of honey-cinnamon drink before and between meals can make you feel full therefore preventing you from snacking in between meals.

In addition, consuming this drink regularly can boost your immune system and also improve your digestive system. It seems like there is no end to what this drink can do. This goes to show just how valuable honey and cinnamon are. Best part is, they come cheap, readily available and generally have no side effects when taken in right proportions.

HONEY FOR HAIR

Honey, when added to hair, smooths the hair follicles, and adds shine to dull hair. This is due to the fact that honey has emollient properties, which is effective for shine and smoothness. Also, the humectants properties in honey bond with water molecules, adding moisture to dry strands. Because honey moisturizes and smooths hair, it enhances the beautiful luster in your hair.

Honey comes highly recommended for hair care. This is because honey has properties that help with cell growth which in turn ensures hair growth. Honey also has the capacity to retain moisture and ameliorate bad scalp conditions such as eczema and dandruff. Simply rub honey into the scalp and hair. Let it sit for twenty minutes then wash off. Do this for a week and you will notice improvements in the hair texture, scalp and general growth.

CHAPTER SIX: PEPPERMINT REMEDIES

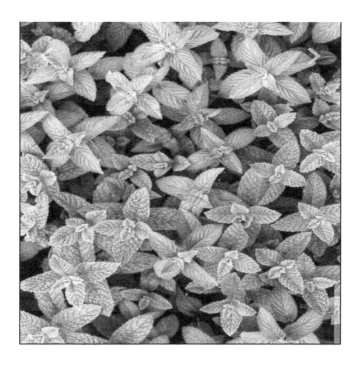

The famous peppermint is a cross between watermint and spearmint. The peppermint essential oil which is extracted from the plant through the means of steam distillation can be used to treat various ailments. The oil has anti-microbial, anti-inflammatory, and antiseptic properties hence it can be used to treat wounds.

Peppermint leaves contain different essential oils including menthol, limonene and menthone. Menthol is what gives peppermint its cooling properties and the cause of its famous minty scent.

This herb is used as flavoring in toothpastes, meals, chewing gum, aromatic candles, candies and other products. The peppermint has soothing effects on people – both physically and emotionally. Peppermint can also be used to treat nausea, menstrual cramps, the common cold, sinus infections, itching, muscle pains, joint pains, indigestion and irritable bowel syndrome (IBS).

In addition to all these, if you are studying for an exam or doing anything that requires a high level of concentration, simply add peppermint essential oil to your diffusers in the room to improve your concentration level, memory and accuracy. It is believed that the peppermint aroma helps with concentration, enhances memory and increases alertness.

You can also apply to the back of the neck and shoulders repeatedly to keep energy levels up during the day. Inhale before and during a workout to help boost your mood and reduce fatigue.

Peppermint essential oil is also used to battle bug problems in the home. Add 5 to 10 drops of essential oil per ounce of warm water, pour this mixture in a spray bottle and spray in areas the bugs stay in. This spray effectively repels bugs.

People with congested sinuses are often told to do a face steaming with peppermint essential oil. This is effective in clearing blocked sinus, relieving cold and lung congestion.

The wonders of this miracle plant do not end there. The peppermint oil helps with hair growth. After a month of regular use, you will notice significant hair growth.

Peppermint oil prevents smooth muscles in the body from contracting. Instead, it relaxes the muscles. That is how it helps with workouts, menstrual cramps and digestive system. Peppermint oil is also effective for toothache as its menthol content has antibacterial properties. Coupled with the cooling properties of the same menthol, this oil gives immediate relief to toothache and heals the guns after days of use.

Please note that the peppermint oil is even more intense than other essential oils so it is advisable to dilute it in a carrier oil like coconut, olive or jojoba oil before topical application. Do not directly apply on the skin to avoid harsh reactions.

Due to all its well-known functions and , the peppermint is high on the list of herbal medicine.

These are some of the uses of the peppermint:

PEPPERMINT OIL FOR COLD

Peppermint relaxes muscles in the windpipe. Its menthol properties soothes an itchy throat. Menthol is a natural decongestant. It softens thick mucus and helps drain the sinus. Menthol is used in most cough medicine in order to soothe the throat.

PEPPERMINT OIL FOR JOINT PAIN

Peppermint has analgesic, antispasmodic, and anti-inflammatory properties. These properties help soothe sore joints. You can put this oil in your bath, or use the essential oil for massage. You can make a cold or hot compress to put pressure on the joints. Simply add the oil to the cold or hot water, immerse the towel, squeeze it and apply on the joints till you feel relief.

PEPPERMINT OIL FOR ITCHY SCALP

Divide the hair into workable parts. Mix peppermint with coconut or jojoba oil and apply directly on the scalp. Then massage the scalp for minutes and rinse after twenty minutes.

Here's how to prepare this hair oil:

- Stir two drops of peppermint oil into one cup of cool water.
- Gently massage the mixture into your scalp for a few minutes.
- Shampoo and condition as usual.

PEPPERMINT OIL FOR SINUS INFECTION

Peppermint opens the trachea and clear sinuses because the menthol affects mucus receptors and fights bacteria.

Menthol may affect the mucus receptors in the nose, helping to open the airway and clear mucus. Lab studies show that peppermint oil may fight bacteria, one of the triggers of sinus congestion.

You can inhale the oil through diffusers, facial steam or add the oil to your hot bath. This should have your sinus cleared within minutes.

PEPPERMINT OIL FOR HEADACHE

Menthol can help relax muscles and ease pain. It's believed that applying diluted peppermint oil topically can help relieve pain from both tension headaches and migraine. Mix peppermint with lavender oil and rub on your forehead for best immediate relief from headaches.

PEPPERMINT OIL FOR FOOT MASSAGE

You can use peppermint for foot soak. It relieves tension in the feet and helps smooth the muscles. Pour two tablespoons of peppermint oil in warm water and soak your feet after a long day or if you have bruises on your feet.

PEPPERMINT FOR NAUSEA

Add peppermint oil to your diffuser when you feel nauseous. You can also add it to hot water for facial steaming. Inhaling peppermint oil relieves nausea. This is because peppermint oil relaxes the gastric muscles and stops them from contracting. You can also chew peppermint gum or lick the mint candy for the same results. Another way of doing this is by drinking peppermint tea.

Here is my peppermint tea recipe:

- Crush peppermint leaves and stem with your hands.
- Boil water.
- Add leaves to boiling water.
- Allow to boil for five minutes.

- Turn off the heat but let the leaves steep for ten minutes.
- Strain the water.
- Add a slice of lemon and a tablespoon of honey.

You can drink this tea for cold, cough and sinus congestion. It is also helpful for indigestion.

PEPPERMINT OIL FOR INDIGESTION

Mix peppermint in a carrier oil and gently massage the abdomen with it. You can also drink peppermint tea for indigestion.

Peppermint helps people with irritable bowel syndrome, or IBS. The properties in peppermint activate an anti-pain channel called TRPM8 in the colon. TRPM8 reduces the pain felt in the body when eating spicy foods.

Orally, you can take coated peppermint oil. Coated oil is advised because though peppermint oil is perfect for indigestion, it can cause heartburns. The coated oil prevents the essential oil from getting in contact with the upper abdomen as the oil gets released from the coating in the small intestine.

PEPPERMINT OIL FOR MENSTRUAL CRAMPS

Mix peppermint oil with a carrier oil and apply topically on the lower abdomen for cramps. This oil increases blood flow, relaxes muscles and stops cramps.

You can also take peppermint tea for similar results. The menthol in the peppermint can help reduce uterine contractions, thereby reducing cramping.

PEPPERMINT OIL FOR TOOTHACHE

Peppermint contains antibacterial properties. These compounds help fight bacterial infection. peppermint oil has been shown to effectively kill bacteria.

It is a proven fact that peppermint reduces several types of bacteria found in the mouth. In addition, menthol has also shown antibacterial activity. Peppermint is also effective for bad breath and other sinus infections.

Rinse the mouth with peppermint water for about a minute. It gives fresher breath, heals sores and prevents the formation of plaque.

PEPPERMINT OIL FOR MEMORY

Inhaling peppermint oil can reduce the effects of Alzheimer's disease. Peppermint improves memory and aids alertness. Add the oil to your diffusers overnight. Or you can put a few drops in hot water and steam.

CHAPTER SEVEN: JASMINE REMEDIES

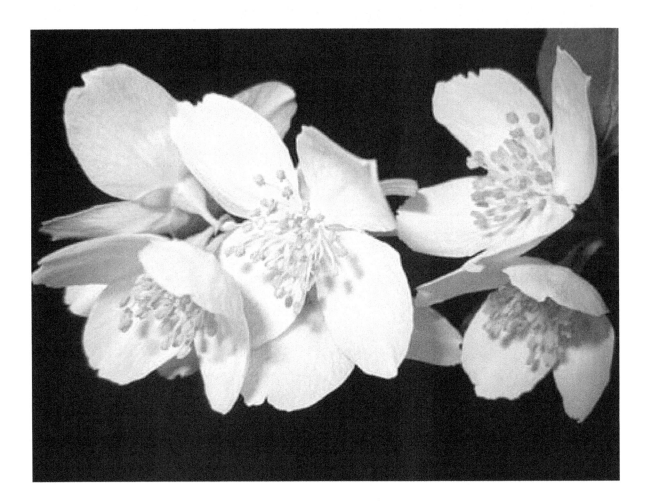

The Jasmine plant, (genus Jasminum) are native to tropical and to some temperate regions of the World. Jasmine are of various types and each type has its own unique purpose and benefits. We have the common Jasmine that is appraised for its aromatic benefits, the Arabian Jasmine lauded for its medicinal tea and many others. Overall, Jasmine continues to play a big role in traditional medicine because of its antioxidants, anticonvulsant, and antidiabetic properties among others. Jasmine is known for preventing seizures, reducing blood sugar and cleansing the body of toxins.

The common jasmine produces scented flowers which are processed into essence for perfumes, soaps, lotions and other beauty products. It is not strange to see Jasmine extract on the labels of your favorite products. Jasmine has been used in some of the most famous scents we know including Chanel No. 5.

The flowers of Arabian Jasmine (which is a jasmine species) are often dried and used to make jasmine tea. The tea is believed to have a lot of medicinal benefits.

Some ailments which respond to Jasmine treatment include: hepatitis, dysentery, seizures, low sexual libido among others. It is also used as treatment for insomnia, and for cancer treatment due to its antitumor properties. Jasmine has been used for hundreds of years in Asia as a natural remedy for depression, emotional stress and low libido.

Its aromatic benefits are numerous and goes from reduction in food cravings to acting as antidepressant. Jasmine scent also acts like an aphrodisiac and also as a sedative. So, this plant works for people with low sex drive and those struggling with mild insomnia.

Jasmine has been proven to have wound healing properties as its extract triggers the process of epithelialization, which is essential for wound closure.

Still, jasmine offers so much more than its powerful fragrance. Jasmine is also used as a flavor for beverages, frozen dairy desserts, candy, baked goods, gelatins, and puddings. All these and much more are packed into this little plant. All you need to do is have some jasmine essential oil or even plant the jasmine in your yard. It's a multipurpose plant and is useful in so many home remedies. What's better? It is generally safe for human use, no preservatives, no chemicals and is all round beneficial.

Listed below are some uses of Jasmine.

JASMINE AS AN APHRODISIAC

Scent is one of the major languages of sexuality. Scent has been a means of arousal and connection between animals since the beginning of time. Scents create powerful, distinctive memories as they serve as a reminder of people and places.

The jasmine scent, when worn by a woman can arouse her partner. Jasmine has a sweet rich scent and is believed to set the sexual mood. So, dab the jasmine oil on your neck, on the inner thighs and beneath the breasts for a heightened sexual ambience. You can also add drops of Jasmine into diffusers to fill the room with the fragrance and create a sexual atmosphere. You can also add a few drops of Jasmine oil to the bath water to give it a sweet scent. Jasmine oil can be used for a romantic massage. There is a big link between touch and sex. Touch of tender massage with the scent of sweet jasmine is the best combination for a romantic night in.

JASMINE AS A PERFUME

You can choose to wear your own jasmine signature scent by creating a special jasmine perfume at home. Follow these steps to make the jasmine perfume:

In a glass container,

- Add 1 tablespoon of distilled water

- 2 tablespoons of vodka
- 35 drops of jasmine
- 5 drops of lavender

Let the mixture sit for at least four weeks in a cool, dark spot. Pour into a glass perfume bottle and your jasmine perfume is ready for use. Note, you can add vanilla or chocolate essence if you want to make a twist.

JASMINE AS AN ANTISEPTIC

Jasmine oil is believed to have antiviral, antibiotic and antifungal properties that makes it effective for boosting immunity and fighting illness. In fact, jasmine has been used to fight candida effectively.

Jasmine has antibacterial properties and can be effectively used to cure bacterial infections on the skin such as eczema, dryness, ringworm etc. Jasmine rejuvenates skins and assists in cell growth. Jasmine is known to have wound healing properties so it can be used as a natural remedy for wound healing.

JASMINE FOR RESTFUL sleep

Jasmine's scent affects GABA. GABA is a brain and central nervous system chemical. Its main role is reduction of the levels of excitability throughout the nervous system. The reduction of excitability ends up calming the nerves, soothing anxiety/mild depression, and encourages relaxation of the body. When nerve signals send signals that could induce anxiety, GABA steps in to slow those signals down, which reduces those feelings of anxiety. So many people use GABA dietary supplements to achieve this state of relaxation.

However, jasmine naturally triggers this GABA chemical to work on your body therefore inducing rest. Jasmine does not necessarily make you sleep more but it ensures you sleep well. It eliminates restlessness and some other sleep problems and generally guarantees a good night's rest. Add a few drops of jasmine oil to your diffusers to enjoy a good night's rest. You can have jasmine as a houseplant in your house for similar effects. Jasmine helps with anxiety and antidepressants. What better way to get the best of this plant than to plant it in your home?

JASMINE FOR HAIR

Jasmine oil is especially good for natural hair. If you want to try a DIY for your hair care cabinet, jasmine is the way to go. Not only does this oil heals the scalp due to its antiseptic properties, it also acts as a moisturizer and a sealant for hair. As an antiseptic, jasmine helps to fight dandruff and other diseases on the scalp. Jasmine is known as a hair moisturizer because of how it adds luster to the hair. To get the best effects, mix five drops of Jasmine essential oil in jojoba oil, divide hair into four parts and use the mixture to massage the scalp and hair, working from the middle of the head to the edges. Then cover hair with a bonnet and let the juices nourish the hair overnight or for about five hours. After, wash hair with warm water and feel the difference in texture. The hair will get way softer therefore making it easier to detangle. This is because of the moisturizing properties in jasmine.

JASMINE FOR DEPRESSION

When people talk about using essential oils for depression, jasmine essential oil must make the list. Like already discussed, jasmine helps trigger GABA which reduces anxiety. Jasmine also boosts moods. If you take a walk in a jasmine garden at night you will immediately feel calmer and happier. Little wonder this plant is recommended for its antidepressant's properties. Rub jasmine oil on your skin for better moods and increase in energy levels.

Also, jasmine is often used during post pregnancy periods. This is because it helps with moods and skin. A good body massage with jasmine, or simply soaking in its bathwater or just applying it topically goes a long way to reduce anxiety and also gives a good-looking skin. Jasmine is even said to reduce scarring and stretch marks on the body. Jasmine is also recommended for menopausal women.

CHAPTER EIGHT: TURMERIC REMEDIES

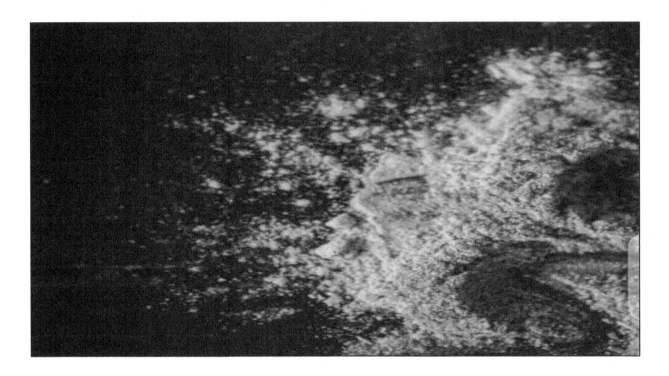

Turmeric is a bright yellow spice obtained from the turmeric plant. It can be recognized by its bright yellow color and pepper-like aroma. Turmeric is not only used in food but also for its medicinal purposes. Turmeric now plays an essential role in the beauty industry, medicine and food.

Turmeric's main content is curcumin and curcumin possesses many bioactivities, such as antioxidant, anti-inflammatory, antiviral, antifungal, cancer chemopreventive, and cancer chemotherapeutic properties. Turmeric is also famous for its benefits to the skin. It rejuvenates the skin by exfoliating dead cells and clearing acne. When paired with eggs and sugar, it is a potent facial scrub. Turmeric face masks are known for bringing out a natural glow. Turmeric organic soap lightens skin, removes spots, blemishes and sunburn.

Due to the presence of its healing properties, turmeric has been used for years to treat many ailments like arthritis, uveitis and even prevents cancer and Alzheimer's disease. It also boosts the immune system. Turmeric is good for the heart and liver. It has been proven through research that turmeric extract reduces markers of liver injury in people who have liver diseases that are not caused by alcohol. Turmeric also helps with fat in the liver as it helps prevent more fat buildup once the ailing person starts taking turmeric. The curcumin in turmeric reduces severe liver injury so it is recommended for people with liver problems to take turmeric with black pepper. This is because black pepper contains piperine which helps in curcumin absorption. Also note that curcumin is fat solvent so you can try to add turmeric whenever you prepare fried meals. The fat breaks down the curcumin for easier absorption in the body. You can make better turmeric tea by mixing turmeric with black pepper and flax oil.

My recipe for this tea is to boil 2 cups of water. Add 2 teaspoons of turmeric. Allow the mixture to simmer for about 10 minutes. Add a tablespoon of black pepper. Add a tablespoon of flax oil. Strain the tea into a container and allow it to cool for 5 minutes. Then serve. You also add a dash of lime or lemon with honey for extra antioxidants and taste. You should begin to notice its effects on your body from four to eight weeks of daily intake.

Turmeric preserves the liver as it prevents alcohol and other toxins from damaging the liver. Note that it is safe to consume turmeric in normal dosages and that too high consumption has side effects.

Turmeric extract is known to help stabilize blood sugar levels and make diabetes more manageable. This can be seen in the fact that the turmeric extract is easily found in many supplements for diabetics. Turmeric also helps in the digestive system as it aids in digestion and prevents constipation. When someone has type 2 diabetes, the body either doesn't produce enough insulin, or it resists insulin. Drinking turmeric root extract helps in reducing insulin resistance that leads to rise in blood sugar levels. It also improves the functioning of beta cells, which are beneficial for diabetes. Also, insulin and triglycerides triggered by high-fat meals can be reduced by a mixture of turmeric and cinnamon tea. This reduction will lead to lower blood sugar levels.

TURMERIC, GINGER AND LEMON FOR NAUSEA

Turmeric, ginger and lemon are super effective for managing nausea. Add a tablespoon spoon of turmeric, a tablespoon of ginger and a squeeze of lemon into boiling water and drink.

TURMERIC AND COCONUT MILK FOR DIABETES

Turmeric being an anti-inflammatory and antioxidant helps to lower blood sugar levels. You can choose to take this daily by adding turmeric to your coconut milk which is another healthy meal.

To make this drink, follow the instructions below:

- Use a hammer to break a coconut.
- Take out the coconut from the shells.
- Blend it with water.
- After blending, pour in a strainer and strain it, squeezing the coconut chaff to get everything out.
- Add a tablespoon of turmeric and a tablespoon of black pepper to it.
- Mix and serve.

TURMERIC FOR WEIGHT LOSS

Turmeric suppresses particular inflammatory markers that play a role in obesity. It has been discovered that there is a link between weight gain and increased inflammation. More weight can mean more inflammation. It is believed that this inflammation may also be a contributing factor that led to the weight gain in the first place. These markers are typically elevated in people with excess weight or obesity. Turmeric has been long known for its anti-inflammatory properties. Therefore, its reduction in the inflammatory markers will result in a reduction in weight. In addition, as an antioxidant, it suppresses the inflammatory condition in pancreatic and fat cells. Some people also say that turmeric curbs cravings which makes them eat less than they used to. Reduction in cravings also leads to weight loss. Also, adding turmeric and chili to hot sauce leads to better metabolism which means more fat burn.

TURMERIC, HONEY AND EGGS FOR FACE MASK.

Turmeric is excellent for skin care as it gives a beautiful glow and supple, calmer skin. Turmeric also lightens skin naturally, clears blemishes, removes dark circles and sunburn, removes dead skin cells and gives a refreshed look.

To make this mask, put 2 tablespoons of turmeric in a bowl, add a tablespoon of honey, crack open an egg and put one egg white in the bowl. Whisk the content until they are well combined. Then apply the mixture on your face and let it sit until it dries. Wash it off with warm water and pat your face with a clean towel.

You can use egg yolk instead of the white. Add one egg yolk, a tablespoon of turmeric and a tablespoon of honey in a bowl. Stir until well incorporated. Then apply on the face till the mixture gets dry. Wash it off with warm water and pat the face dry with a towel.

What to bear in mind when choosing egg white or yolk is that egg whites contain albumin, which is a simple protein for reducing pores and clear blackheads, making them especially great for oily skin. On the other hand, egg yolk moisturizes dry skin as it contains fatty acids and proteins. So, while making your choice you have to take your skin type into consideration. Dry skin Should use egg yolk to moisturize. Oily skin that is prone to acne should make use of egg whites.

TURMERIC, SUGAR AND LEMON FOR BODY SCRUB

Body scrubs are used to exfoliate the skin by removing dead skin cells and replacing them with new ones. Turmeric is filled with antioxidants and anti-inflammatory properties so combining it with brown sugar is superb. Brown sugar contains glycolic acid, an antibacterial and exfoliating agent that keeps acne in check and improves the look and feel of skin. Brown sugar also reduces sunburn and gives a wrinkle free skin. Lemon has a high pH level which decreases the inflammation and the oil on skin. Oil and inflammation contribute to the formation of acne. As a result, lemon juice dries up acne. Furthermore, the citric acid in lemon, a type of alpha hydroxy acid (AHA), can help break down dead skin cells that lead to noninflammatory forms of acne like blackheads.

TURMERIC, ALOE VERA AND CARROT OIL FOR CLEAR SKIN

We have already said turmeric is great for the skin because of its curcumin property. Now aloe vera is also the perfect paste for the skin because of its contents. The aloe vera contain vitamins such as vitamins A, C and E, which are antioxidants. Aloe vera also contains vitamin B12, folic acid, and choline enzymes, minerals, sugars, lignin, saponins, salicylic acids and amino acids. Aloe vera heals wounds, absorbs oil easily, provides quick relief from burning, and cold sores. Due to its anti-inflammatory properties aloe vera can treat acne that occurs as a result of inflammation.

Carrot oil on the other hand is popular in beauty products as it contains beta carotene and vitamin A. It is lauded as anti-aging oil because it rejuvenates, lightens and smooths the skin. It also clears blemishes, acne and offers protection against harsh weather.

Therefore, turmeric, carrot oil and aloe vera mixture can be combined to produce an anti-aging, blemish cleansing, soft and supple facial skin.

You can make this mask at home by following the steps below:

- Break off a leaf of aloe vera, scoop out aloe vera gel into a bowl.
- Add two tablespoons of turmeric.
- Add a tablespoon of carrot oil.
- Whisk till you make a smooth paste.
- Apply this on the face for about twenty minutes.
- Without using soap, wash off with warm water and pat the face dry with a towel.

This paste will keep your skin looking refreshed. After weeks of consistent use, you will notice you have achieved a much younger look.

TURMERIC AND APPLE CIDER VINEGAR FOR WOUNDS

Turmeric has high antiseptic properties which makes it a go to option for wounds. Turmeric's healing properties stop bleeding and prevent the wound from getting infected. Apple cider vinegar has anti itching properties which also helps in wound treatment. If you have a cut, apply turmeric—apple cider vinegar mixture to heal it.

To make the paste:

Mix a tablespoon of turmeric with a tablespoon of apple cider vinegar to make a paste.

Apply this paste in the wound and cover with a gauze. Change this daily till the wound heals.

TURMERIC FOR IMMUNE SYSTEM BOOST.

Curcumin which is found in turmeric boosts the immune system. Also, turmeric has lipopolysaccharides and endotoxins. These properties boost immunity and lower the risk of getting infected with minor diseases. Daily turmeric intake helps to protect one against some minor infections like the common cold.

TURMERIC AND CANCER

Turmeric contains curcumin which is known for its anti-cancer effects. Research has shown lower rates of certain cancers in countries where people eat more curcumin. The level of curcumin needed is about 100mg to 200mg a day over long periods of time.

Curcumin has the capacity to kill cancer cells and even prevent more from growing therefore slowing the disease's progression. It has been seen to have the best effects on preventing breast cancer, bowel cancer, stomach cancer and skin cancer cells. You can add turmeric to your meals, make its tea or apply topically on cancerous spots when it pertains to skin cancer.

TURMERIC AND MEMORY

Curcumin improves memory and mood in older people. Turmeric powder may diminish beta-amyloid plaques in the brain because of its curcumin content. This means that turmeric is helpful in treating Alzheimer's disease.

CHAPTER NINE: ALOE VERA REMEDIES

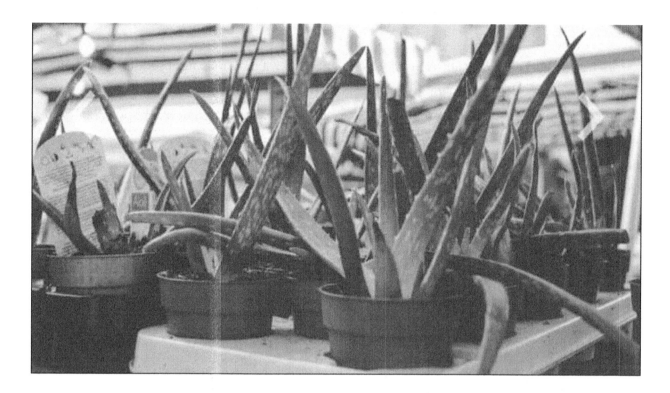

Aloe vera, though considered a tropical plant, had been used by Native Americans for its medicinal purposes which was mainly to soothe and heal the skin. Today, the aloe vera is grown in every part of the world. Aloe vera is a shrub with thick leaves.

Aloe vera leaf has three main layers. The inner layer is a gel with water content that goes as high as 99%, and the remaining part is made of amino acids, glucomannans, sterols, lipids, and vitamins. The middle layer is made of latex, which is a yellow sap containing glycosides and anthraquinones.

Because of its medicinal properties, aloe vera is considered one of the most highly rated herbal plants in America. This wonder plant has been used to treat various ailments ranging from skin diseases, to lowering of blood sugar and also serve as a substitute mouthwash.

Apart from healing the human body, aloe vera can also be used to keep other produce fresh for a long period of time. It has been noted that apples which are coated with aloe vera gel stay fresher for longer periods than those that are not. This also proved to be true for other fruits and vegetables. So, we can safely say that aloe vera gel contains a compound that preserves freshness. Due to the fact that aloe vera contains antibacterial compounds, coating any produce with aloe vera gel stops the growth of harmful bacteria.

The aloe vera has antiviral, antibacterial and antifungal properties. The bioactive compounds in aloe vera helps fight against skin diseases, ulcer, diabetes, dysentery and other numerous ailments.

Aloe vera can be taken orally or applied topically. The gel can be applied directly on the skin to treat wounds, dryness and other skin diseases. It can be added to tea and foods in order to treat digestive problems or other internal ailments. Aloe vera is generally safe for human consumption but if you have any underlying ailment, talk to your doctor before you start aloe vera treatment. It also goes without saying that if you're allergic to aloe vera you should avoid this.

Apart from taking this herb to heal diseases aloe vera is also one of the top natural products for skin care. It is found in makeup, soap, perfume, lotion, shampoo, hair cream and other skin care products. Aloe vera serves as a moisturizer to the skin. Aloe vera improves skin tone, removes sunburn and black spots. It also clears the skin of blemishes, dries pimples and generally lightens the skin. Due to the presence of antioxidants and vitamins, aloe vera protects the skin from UV rays of the sun. It also helps free the face of wrinkles and fine lines. It is a good source of sunscreen so it is used in various over-the-counter sunscreen products. You can use aloe vera gel for your natural sunscreen remedy at home. The high water content serves to hydrate and moisturize your skin. The antibacterial contents prevent the skin from overexposure to the sun.

It helps with dry skin and nourishes natural hair as it is known for enhancing hair growth, reducing dandruff and healing the scalp of eczema.

We will state below some of the uses of aloe vera in natural remedies and the other products aloe vera can be combined with to give excellent results.

ALOE VERA FACIAL MASKS

Aloe vera has a high number of mucopolysaccharides, a hydrating molecule that keeps moisture in the skin. Aloe also releases fibroblasts which heightens collagen production and elastin fibers. Collagen is the reason for your body's elasticity. But as one grows older, it gets harder for the body to produce collagen therefore limiting flexibility. Aloe vera activates the production of collagen which keeps the body flexible with better joints, supple skin and minimal wrinkles.

Aloe vera is rich in vitamins and water so it naturally hydrates and moisturizes the skin. It also lightens the skin pigmentation. Little wonder that aloe vera is the base for many skin care products. For a home remedy, mix aloe vera with honey and lemon. Lemon is antibacterial and also has lightening properties.

To obtain the aloe vera face mask,

- Mix aloe vera gel in a plate
- Add two tablespoons of lemon and a tablespoon of honey.
- Stir till they are well combined.
- Apply this mask on the face and leave it to dry.
- Once it dries off wash your face with warm water and pat it dry with a towel. You should see results in a week of this daily regimen.

ALOE VERA AND HONEY LOTION

Add aloe vera and honey to your body lotion to better moisturize your skin.

Take two tablespoons of aloe vera gel and mix with 2 tablespoons of raw honey.

Add the mixture to your body lotion.

Shake the lotion container until it is well incorporated, then use the lotion as usual.

ALOE VERA FOR HAIR

You can add aloe vera to your shampoo and conditioner. You simply mix it in those products and use them as usual. Aloe vera is good for hair growth as its antibacterial and antiseptic compounds work to heal the scalp of dandruff, dryness, eczema and other infections. Aloe vera also moisturizes the scalp, nourishes the hair with vitamins which ensures hair growth. Apart from adding aloe vera to your shampoo, you can make aloe vera masks for your hair.

Mix aloe vera with honey and jojoba oil and apply generously to your scalp and hair at night. After application, cover your hair with a bonnet and go to bed. Wash it out the next day and you will notice that your hair is softer and has more shine. Do this regularly and your hair will grow better faster with a noticeable reduction in hair breakage.

For people with itchy scalp, mix aloe vera gel with mint oil and grated ginger or ginger oil and apply to your hair. Let it sit for 20 minutes before you wash it out. Repeat this thrice a week for best results.

ALOE VERA, BEETROOT AND HONEY FOR LIPS

Aloe vera contains aloesin, a flavonoid that makes lips pink. It also contains moisturizer that keeps lips hydrated and soft. Beetroot adds a natural pink shade on skin when applied over a period of time. Honey moisturizes the lips. So, making this together for your special lip balm is going to ensure you have rosy pink lips. To make this special balm, mix aloe vera gel in a bowl, add a teaspoon of beetroot juice then add a teaspoon of honey. Apply this mixture on your lips overnight for best results. You should notice a difference after a week of daily use. You can keep this balm in the freezer to harden it up or mix with your old lipstick.

You can also use aloe vera as scrub to exfoliate the lips. Put two tablespoons of aloe vera gel in a bowl, add a tablespoon of brown sugar, a tablespoon of beetroot juice and mix this together. Then use your toothbrush to pack the mixture and gently scrub your lips with it for a few minutes. This will exfoliate your lips and give it a beautiful pink hue.

ALOE VERA AND DENTAL HEALTH

Aloe vera has antibacterial, antifungal and anti-inflammatory properties. These compounds help prevent plague in the mouth and hastens the healing process of dental diseases. Aloe vera mouthwash gives fresh breath and stronger gums. It also reduces plague drastically. Aloe vera can be used to treat other mouth infections like cold sores, canker sores etc. Its antibacterial and antiseptic properties help to heal wounds in the mouth.

To get this natural remedy simply extract aloe vera gel into a bowl, add mint essential oil, mix them together and use it to brush just before you go to bed at night. Also gargle aloe vera and mint water after each meal.

ALOE VERA FOR DIABETES

Taking two tablespoons of aloe vera daily can lower blood sugar. Aloe vera has the capacity to lower blood sugar and increase the good glucose in the human body. The best part is, aloe vera is cheap, contains no preservatives and generally has no side effects. You can drink aloe vera as a smoothie, tea or cocktail.

To make a smoothie, put aloe vera in a blender, add half a lime, and one cucumber. Blend until smooth. Serve immediately.

ALOE VERA FOR DIGESTION AND HEARTBURN

Taking aloe vera just before meals helps with heart burns because of the plant's low toxicity levels. Aloe vera is a gentler, better and cheaper medicine for heartburn and digestion problems.

Here are some ways to take aloe vera:

- You can take aloe vera in other smoothies.
- You can blend it and drink pure aloe vera juice.
- You can add it to cocktails and drink.
- You can also make aloe vera tea and drink whenever you want.

To make aloe vera tea take two tablespoons of aloe vera gel plus a tablespoon of mint oil, pour them into a glass of water and bring it to boil. Your aloe vera tea is ready.

CHAPTER TEN: BEETROOT REMEDIES

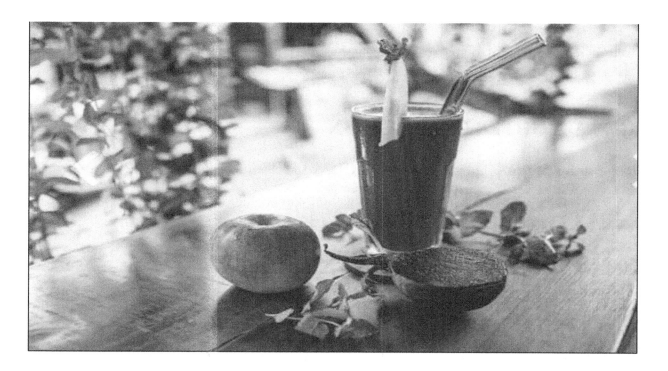

Beetroot, which is also known as red beet, table beet, garden beet, or simply beet, is a root vegetable filled with so many essential nutrients. The beetroot is excellent in helping lower blood pressure for those suffering from high blood pressure. It also fights inflammation; this is because the beetroot contains anti-inflammatory properties.

Beetroot contains vitamin c which helps the skin maintain its elasticity and slows down the aging process. Taking beetroots regularly can boost your brainpower and increase exercise stamina.

Beetroot betalains effectively prevent colon cancer. The fibrous contents of beetroots ease bowel movements which reduces the time that stool spends in the intestines, thereby minimizing the colon's exposure to potential carcinogens.

Beetroot has skin lightening properties so it lightens dark lips. Also, its red color turns dark lips to a rosy pink.

BEETROOT FOR PINK LIPS

- Mix a tablespoon of beetroot with a tablespoon of honey and apply on the lips.
- Let it sit for twenty minutes.
- Wash it off after that.

You can also apply and allow it sit overnight. The honey will heal the lips of cracks and removes deaf cells. The beetroot lightens and add a pink hue to the lips.

BEETROOT FOR HAIR

Cut beetroot in half and scrub on the scalp. The juice will seep in and moisturize the scalp. It will also nourish the hair and allow it to grow fuller and better.

To GET A LIGHTER COMPLEXION

Beetroot contains vitamin C and we know vitamin C helps in collagen production in the body.

Lemon juice on the other hand, is one of the top natural skin brightening agents. Lemon helps in providing an even tone to your skin by clearing blemishes and dark spots.

To make this beetroot and lemon mask, you need:

- 1 tablespoon of beetroot juice
- 1 tablespoon of lemon juice

Preparation:

- In a bowl, mix both the ingredients.
- Apply the mixture on your face.
- Leave it on for 15 minutes.
- Rinse it off later.
- Pat the face dry with a clean towel.

CHAPTER ELEVEN: LEMONGRASS REMEDIES

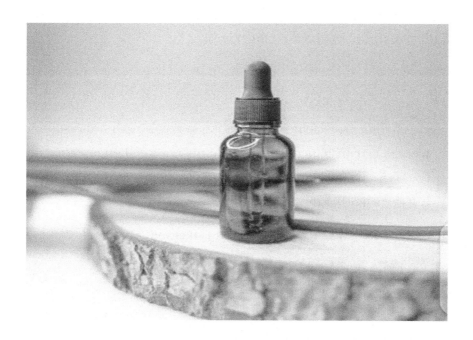

Lemongrass contains antibacterial and antifungal properties, which help prevent or kill harmful bacteria. It also contains properties that can help fight against fever or lower levels of sugar cholesterol. It prevents infection because of its antibacterial properties. Lemongrass is good for the liver as it lowers the enzyme activity and stress in the liver.

Furthermore, lemongrass increases metabolism. Now metabolism is the chemical reaction in our bodies that changes food to energy, hence, aids weight loss. So, drinking lemongrass helps in shedding that extra weight. In addition, lemongrass can be used to treat problems in the digestive tract, high blood pressure convulsions, rheumatism, common cold, and exhaustion. Lemongrass is also a mild sedative, as its smell can lull you to sleep. So, the fragrance is perfect for bedtime slumber. The oil is packed with vitamin A, C, and limonene, which lighten skin, so bathing with lemongrass homemade soap or lemongrass lotion can lighten the skin. Lemongrass has purifying substances which help detoxify the skin. This property removes impurities from your skin, cleans up, opens up your pores, takes away dead cells, and rejuvenates your skin to give you a brighter Sheen.

Add lemongrass regularly to your bath water or use it as an oil to get clearer skin. You can also use lemongrass to treat an itchy scalp because of its antifungal element. Furthermore, lemongrass thickens hair as it strengthens the hair follicles, therefore, allowing hair to grow better.

In addition to all these benefits, lemongrass acts as a potent mosquito repellent because mosquitoes cannot stand the smell of lemongrass. You could put this in your diffusers to repel mosquitoes. Pure lemon oil can be diffused for calmness as it has properties that eliminate anxiety and eliminate fatigue.

To use lemongrass oil, you should add it to a carrier oil to dilute it, as undiluted lemongrass oil can be harsh on the skin. Once it's diluted, the oil can be used for skincare.

Another way to use lemongrass is to boil in a pot. Once it boils, pour it into a bowl, put your face above it, cover your head with thick clothing and inhale the steam for malaria fever or the common cold.

Lemongrass is also used as a diuretic, which means that it is used to expel urine and salt from the body as a form of treatment. People with certain ailments who take lemongrass end up urinating more and expelling salt from their bodies, thereby cleansing the kidney through the use of lemongrass. Since lemongrass is a diuretic, it can help in weight loss by expelling fats from your body.

It is also believed that lemongrass cures malaria through this method.

Some of the ways to incorporate lemongrass into your lifestyle are by taking its tea and by steaming. Here are some natural remedies one can do with lemongrass.

LEMONGRASS FOR NERVOUSNESS

Lemongrass is effective for nervousness. Add lemongrass oil to diffuser or sip lemongrass tea to calm the nerves.

LEMONGRASS FOR MALARIA

For hundreds of years, Africans have used lemongrass to treat fever. In fact, in some regions in West Africa, lemongrass is known as the fever grass. The grass is boiled in a big pot. Once it's boiled, the pot is placed on the ground and a stool kept in front of it. The person suffering from malaria is then given a stick to rapidly turn the contents of the pot in order to release vapor. A thick blanket is placed over the person and the hot pot for about 10 minutes. A cup of the lemongrass water is given to the person to drink. After the exercise, the person washes all the sweat away and immediately the fever goes away with the sweat.

LEMONGRASS FOR YEAST INFECTION

Lemongrass has antifungal properties. Examples of Fungi are yeast and mold. Lemongrass oil is an effective deterrent against some kinds of fungi.

LEMONGRASS FOR ANXIETY

Lemongrass reduces anxiety. To lift your mood, you either put the oil in your diffusers or you can rub the oil on your body to bring on a calming effect.

CHAPTER TWELVE: THYME REMEDIES

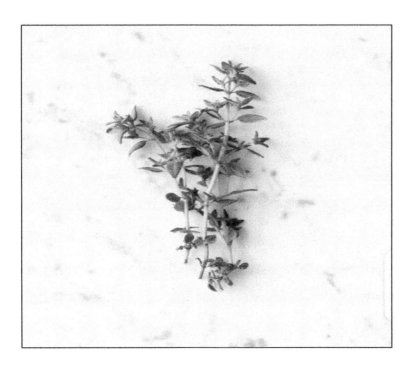

Thyme is an aromatic herb that is not only used for culinary purposes but its medicinal benefits. Due to its antifungal, anti-inflammatory, and anti-bacterial properties is used as a preservative in food. Thyme cures bronchitis, whooping cough, arthritis, stomach pain, flatulence, coughs and other upper respiratory diseases.

Thyme is a useful herb that can help with cough as it has a spasmolytic effect on smooth muscle, meaning it can help relax tight muscles. This is especially important with asthma.

You can use it during nasal congestion to drain mucus and decongest the nose. Using thyme to drain mucus is pretty easy.

- Add thyme to boiling water and let it simmer for 10 minutes.
- Pour into a bowl and put your face over it to inhale the steam.
- Inhale for about 5 minutes.

The thyme will open your airway, soften mucus and allow it to drain out easily, therefore, decongesting the trachea.

This powerful herb can also boost your immune system as it is a good source of iron, copper, and other important immune system boosters.

Flavonoids are a compound found in thyme. This property relaxes the muscles involved in coughing and also reduces inflammation.

CHAPTER THIRTEEN: FENUGREEK REMEDIES

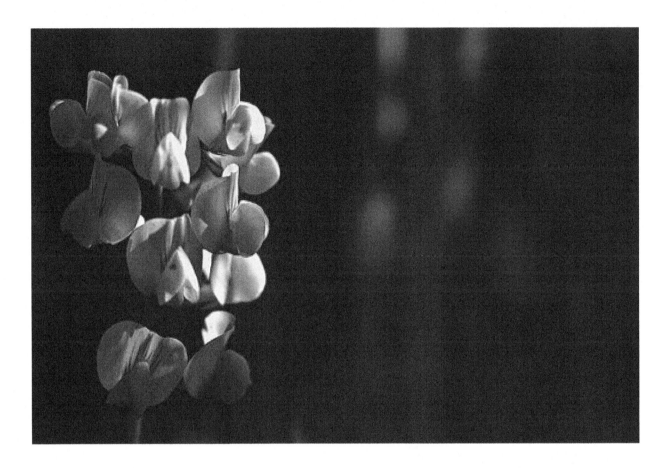

Fenugreek helps with digestion, breast milk production, diabetes, menopause, painful menstruation, breathing problems, labor pains, increase in breast and buttocks, low libido, erectile dysfunction and lots more.

Fenugreek is a remedy used to increase the production of breast milk. Most people believe that fenugreek boosts milk production in women.

Fenugreek is also used to induce labor and treat urinary tract problems.

Fenugreek has always been used to treat skin problems. Fenugreek also controls diabetes and blood sugar levels. It also reduces triglycerides and bad cholesterol levels.

Fenugreek helps people to grow bigger buttocks, as the natural hormones in fenugreek helps to promote estrogen production. This means that you can use fenugreek to grow your buttocks, hips and breasts naturally. What triggers the estrogens is a special component known as diosgenin. Also, fenugreek has phytoestrogens which are more like the human estrogens that regulate hormones.

Fenugreek also enhances bowel movement as it has properties that battles constipation. Fenugreek is also great for hair.

Fenugreek for Breast Enlargement

Mix fenugreek oil with marker oil and warm the mixture on a stove. Then dip your fingers into the mixture and move your fingers around for a massage. You should notice an increase in buttocks size after three weeks of daily massage.

FENUGREEK FOR LOWER BLOOD SUGAR

Fenugreek significantly reduces blood sugar and helps with insulin response. The fibrous seeds slow the body's absorption of carbohydrates and sugar. It also increases the good cholesterol and reduces the bad ones. Fenugreek also helps prevent diabetes as it's been shown that people who take fenugreek regularly are less likely to develop diabetes.

Put two tablespoons of fenugreek seeds in a kettle with a glass of water and boil for 15 minutes. Strain the tea out. Add honey and serve. Drink this tea first thing in the morning daily.

Fenugreek for Breast Milk

Fenugreek has been proven to aid lactation in women who find it difficult to produce enough breast milk for their infants. Drinking fenugreek triggers the production of breast milk. To take this for lactation, you have to prepare the fenugreek tea. Follow these steps to make the tea.

- Wash the fenugreek seeds
- Put the seeds in a pot add water and boil
- Strain the seeds and serve tea hot.
- You can add honey, sugar or any sweetener to the tea.

CHAPTER FOURTEEN: LEMON REMEDIES

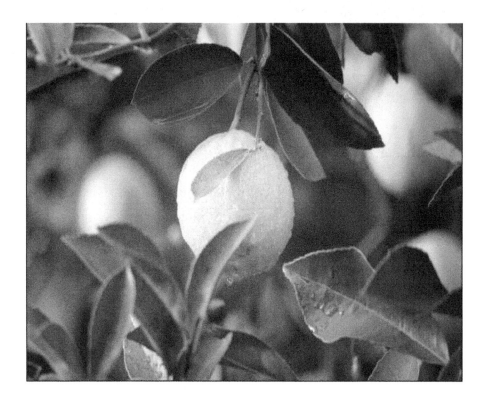

Lemon is a fruit in the citrus family. Lemon has many health benefits and supports weight loss, prevents skin diseases, protects against anemia, and helps with digestive tract issues. Lemon also provides hydration and improves skin quality, freshens breath, and cures many diseases because of its anti-inflammatory properties.

In addition, lemon is known to fight respiratory diseases, sore throat, and inflammation of the tonsils. Lemon leaves help rid the vagina of odor. Also, lemon increases collagen in the body, which means that you will have fewer wrinkles and clear skin if you drink lemon water.

Drinking lemon water in the morning energizes the body, so, taking a glass of warm lemon water 30 minutes before meals helps to curb appetite and also helps in digestion and reduction of heartburn and bloating. It also helps flush toxins in the digestive tract. Lemon water serves to uplift the mood, cure anxiety, and reduce depression. Consistent taking of lemon water lightens the complexion and helps with weight loss as it reduces bloating due to the fact that lemon is a natural diuretic that cleanses the body of extra salt and therefore reduces bloating. In addition, drinking lemon in hot water reduces joint pain, healthy toothaches, and prevents gingivitis. Apart from lightening the skin, lemon can clear the skin of acne and pimples. It is also effective for dandruff. Lemon is also good for the kidney as it contains citrate, which prevents the buildup of calcium, resulting in the formation of stones in the kidney.

Lemon oil also reduces morning sickness in pregnant women. Put three drops of lemon oil in your diffuser overnight for best results. Or drink lemon tea first thing in the morning. You can also put the oil in a carrier oil like carrot oil and apply it to the face. Doing this reduces morning sickness as lemon oil has nausea-fighting properties.

Lemon being antibacterial, kills bacteria in pores which prevent pimples and acne. Due to its antioxidant properties, lemon oil also clears blackheads, acne, and other skin blemishes. Because of its vitamin c, lemon oil exfoliates dead cells that are in hair follicles which helps the body produce thicker hair. Mix lemon oil and apply thoroughly to the scalp.

The vitamin c in Lemon boosts immunity, so taking a glass of lemon water daily can boost your immune system. This triggers your white blood cells to fight diseases and also helps with blood circulation.

Lemon is not only good for whitening skin, it is also a good cleaning agent as it cleanses ceramic surfaces and other surfaces in the home.

You can use lemon to clean your food like fish, shrimp, whiten rice, etc. Lemon has antibacterial properties, so it kills bacteria in food. You can add lemon to the water used in washing fruits.

Lemon is a disinfectant, so it can be used to clean the bathroom, kitchen and to wash dishes. to remove tough stains from ceramic and tiles and to freshen the refrigerator. Adding lemon juice with vinegar juice makes the best homemade cleaning agents. The lemon juice acts as bleach because of its antiseptic and antibacterial content. It is very simple to use lemon in cleaning. Simply cut the lemon in half and use it to scrub sink, washbasin, and other tough stains.

You can add it to your bathing water for a fresher feel and to toothpaste for healthier gums, fresher breath, and whiter teeth. Lemon can also be used as a mild deodorant.

Lemon is one of the best air fresheners as it eliminates foul odor in the home and leaves a lemony fresh air. Lemon is also good for relieving stress, so if you cut a slice of lemon into a plate and keep it next to your bed, it opens your airways and allows you to sleep more easily as it kills toxins in the air.

It is ridiculously easy to make a lemon cleaner. All you need is 4 cups of vodka, half cup of white vinegar, half cup of lemon juice, a cup of water and 4 cups of hydrogen peroxide, and one tablespoon of liquid castile soap. Mix these together, then keep them in a cool dark place for 48 hours. Shake and use.

Because lemon has been said to uplift mood, cure anxiety, and lower depression, add lemon oil to your diffuser overnight. This oil will improve your mood, energize you and reduce depression. Also add the oil to your cream or your shower gel as it is capable of lifting your moods. You can even add lemon to your air freshener cans to give them a fresher smell.

Lemon kills germs, so lemon tea is highly effective for the common cold, cough, and other respiratory problems. To make your lemon tea, boil a glass of water, add ginger strain and serve, squeeze a lemon, and add a tablespoon of honey and drink..

CONCLUSION

As you have seen, natural remedies can be very effective at battling ailment and maintaining wholeness. The advice here is subject to your doctor's advice as your doctor alone can properly advise you based on your personal diagnosis and medical history. Most of the remedies here are generally safe with little to no side effects, but due to individual differences and underlying medical issues, the remedies here are subject to your doctor's professional counsel.

The good part about natural remedies is the absence of additives, preservatives and the freshness of the products used. Part of the advantages is the certainty of knowing that you are taking these things in their pure forms, not adulterated fixes. Due to the high rate of chemically manufactured medication, this book was written to help people access natural remedies to prevent ailments that could cost them thousands of dollars to treat.

Ensure that you take the natural herbs discussed in this book in their correct dosage. Many people think that natural remedies cannot be abused or overdosed. That is false information. Even natural herbs can be abused, so always stick to the right dosage. If it does not work, see your doctor. Also, it is worthy of note that being natural and mild may take a longer time to see results. So, you have to be patient, consistent, and stick to the proper dosage to achieve what you are looking for. You can also research other uses of the herbs in this book and herbs that have not been mentioned in this book.

BOOK 5
NATURAL REMEDIES
FOR CHILDREN

CHAPTER ONE: ARE HERBAL REMEDIES SAFE FOR CHILDREN?

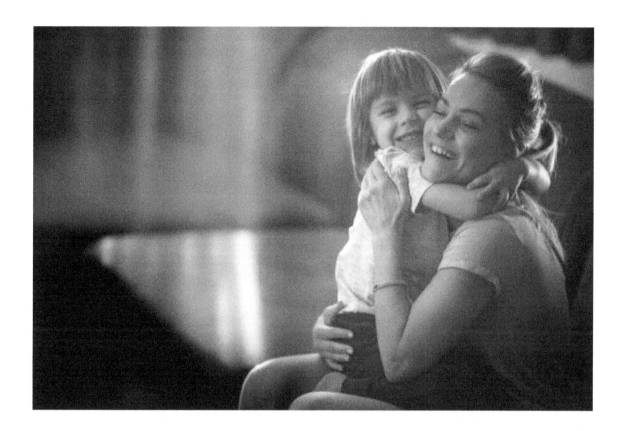

Medicine is incredibly important to us human beings. Medical advancements have allowed doctors to heal various types of illnesses, sicknesses, and diseases, and it has allowed them to save countless lives. All parents want their children to receive the highest quality medical care, and, as such, it is also every child's right to receive it. However, it is quite evident that high-quality medical care is expensive. So, is there a way to get it at a lower cost but with the same amount of safety and effectiveness?

Nowadays, medicine can be obtained from a variety of sources. Although they are commonly made in laboratories by mixing chemicals together, organisms can also be used to create medicine such as penicillin which is a byproduct of fungus. Other types of medicines are made from plants, or medicinal herbs, which have been used for as long as can be remembered – and which are still used by parents all over the world today.

Only a few parents are aware of the existence and benefits of natural, herbal remedies used in treating a variety of health issues present in most children. Certain plants' roots, stems, leaves, flowers, seeds, and even berries can be used to create these herbal remedies. They can be turned into powders, tinctures, tea, ointments, and salves. Aside from herbs, spices can be used to create homemade, natural remedies that will surely help lessen the symptoms of most minor illnesses.

Most herbal remedies are safe. According to Craig Hospital, at least 80% of the world's population incorporates medicinal herbs in their healthcare. Of course, this doesn't mean that you should give your child herbal or natural remedies exclusively. As a rule of thumb, you should be cautious when giving your child any type of medication.

When using medicinal herbs, make sure your child isn't allergic to any of them. This can be done by doing a patch test. Simply take a bit of the herb you plan to use in your child's remedy and apply it to their skin. If it causes a negative reaction, do NOT use that herb. If it does not cause any negative reactions, you should still only incorporate small amounts at a time to be completely sure. You should also make certain to inform your child's physician or doctor about any changes and additions you make in your child's diet or medicinal intake.

CHAPTER TWO: SAFE DOSAGE FOR CHILDREN

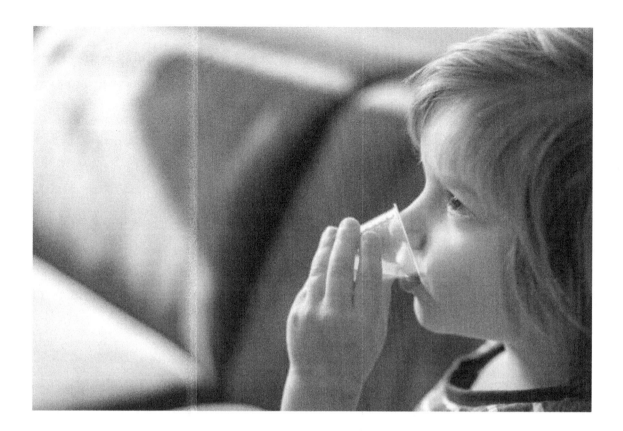

Tea

Teas are helpful in curing minor illnesses and issues like an upset stomach, nausea, sore throat, and even anxiety. They can help calm and relax children, especially if they are having trouble sleeping. They are also a wonderful, hydrating alternative to soft drinks and juice, especially if the tea is made from fruits like raspberry, blueberry, or peach.

Herbal teas like peppermint, chamomile, and fruit tea do not contain caffeine, unlike black or green tea. This means it is completely safe for children to drink them if they are given the proper amount.

- For children younger than 2 years old, the recommended dosage of tea is ½ - 1 teaspoon
- For children aged between 2 to 4 years old, the recommended dosage of tea is 2 teaspoons
- For children aged between 4 to 7 years old, the recommended dosage of tea is 1 tablespoon
- For children aged between 7 to 12 years old, the recommended dosage of tea is 2 tablespoons
- For children aged over 12, the recommended dosage of tea is 1 cup or 8 oz

Tincture

A tincture dropperful, or a squeeze, is the amount of liquid that fills the glass tube of a dropper. Sometimes, the liquid won't fill the glass tube fully, however, that is still considered as a dropperful or approximately 30 drops.

Tinctures are often used by people who don't have enough time or have no love for brewing herbs to make medicine. Tinctures can also be used to make tea instantly by simply adding 2 droppersful into a cup of warm water. They are also easier to give to children as only small amounts are given at a time.

- For children aged 2 to 3 years old, the recommended dosage of tincture is 10 drops
- For children aged 3 to 4 years old, the recommended dosage of tincture is 12 drops
- For children aged between 4 to 6 years old, the recommended dosage of tincture is 15 drops
- For children aged between 6 to 9 years old, the recommended dosage of tincture is 24 drops
- For children aged between 9 to 12 years old, the recommended dosage of tincture is 30 drops or 1 dropperful
- For children aged over 12, the recommended dosage of tincture is 60 drops or 2 droppersful

Other Ways to Determine the Recommended Dosage

If the remedy you want to give your child isn't in the form of a tea or tincture, there are other ways to determine a child's recommended dosage. The most popular ways are Young's Rule and Cowling's Rule. They are both methods of calculation to determine the recommended safe dosage for children.

Young's Rule

- Add 12 to the child's age.
- Divide the child's age by this total.
- Get the recommended dosage for the child

For example, the dosage for a 6-year-old child would be: 6 divided by 18 (6 + 12) = 0.33 or ⅓ of an adult's dosage.

Cowling's Rule

- Divide the number of the child's next birthday by 24.
- Get the recommended dosage for the child.

For example, the dosage for a child who is 5, turning 6 would be: 6 divided by 24 = 0.25 or ¼ of an adult's dosage.

CHAPTER THREE: COMMON HEALTH ISSUES EXPERIENCED BY CHILDREN

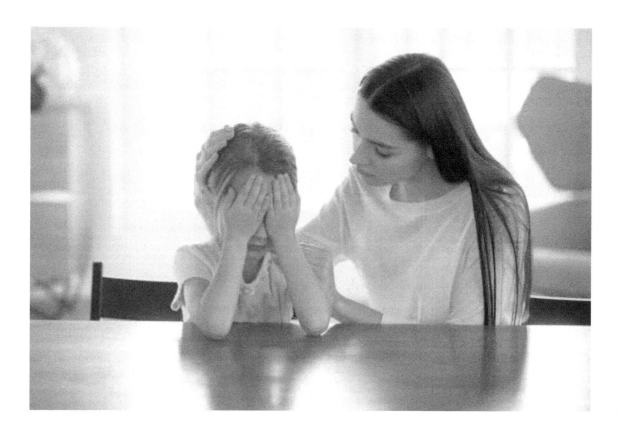

Eczema

Eczema is a skin condition that can appear in adults as well as children. It is characterized by dry patches appearing on the skin. It is itchy and uncomfortable. This skin condition can present itself in children with a family history of eczema, allergies, hay fever, or even asthma. It can be triggered by small irritants such as a particular type of fabric like wool, soap, or detergent, and = environmental factors like humidity and heat. It can also be triggered by various allergens like food, dust, or pollen.

Symptoms Of Eczema

Eczema may appear as reddish, brownish-gray patches on hands, feet, neck, chest, elbows, knees, and (for babies) on the face and scalp. Children with eczema may also have thick, cracked, scaly skin that severely itches, especially at night. Eczema can also cause small bumps to appear on the skin, which can leak fluid and crust over once scratched.

How To Prevent Eczema

There isn't a specific way to prevent eczema, but one of the best ways is to avoid being in contact with anything that triggers or flares up your child's eczema. Another way is to help your child by ensuring their skin isn't too dry as it can cause itchiness which can worsen their condition. You can also use unscented soaps or non-soap cleansers when giving them short baths in warm water.

When To See a Doctor

- Itchiness is so severe that it affects you or your child's daily activities
- When your child appears to have red streaks, pus, or yellow scabs on their skin – this may become a skin infection

If your child appears to have a fever or skin infection, immediately seek medical attention from a doctor.

Insomnia

Insomnia is described as difficulty in falling asleep, staying asleep, or going back to sleep. While adults are more likely to have trouble sleeping, insomnia can also be experienced by children. This can be caused by many factors, most of which are often due to their daytime habits. Children who watch too much television and eat a lot of sugary foods often have difficulty going to bed at night. They are also prone to getting night terrors or bedtime fears.

Symptoms Of Insomnia

Children with insomnia can appear cranky, irritable, and absent-minded, or spaced out. They can also appear visibly tired during the day (daytime sleepiness or drowsiness). They often make mistakes and have trouble remembering things they are supposed to remember.

How To Prevent Insomnia

To prevent your child from having insomnia, you can decrease the amount of time your child spends in front of the TV. You can also reduce their sugar consumption. Try doing activities during the day that will tire them out, so they will be tired enough to sleep through the night. Also, make sure they are comfortable in their room or bed.

When To See a Doctor

- Extreme difficulty doing daytime activities

- If trouble sleeping persists for more than a few days or a week
- If insomnia continues even after healthy changes in the child's lifestyle have been applied

Occasional insomnia isn't necessarily a bad thing. However, when your child often gets less than the required and necessary hours of sleep time they should be getting, you should consult a doctor or a sleep specialist as soon as possible.

Constipation

Constipation is the difficulty in pooping, and it is often experienced by infants when they first start eating solid food, toddlers when they first begin potty training, and older children when they first start school. It is often caused by a lack of fiber intake and fluids. Some medications can also cause constipation. This in turn leads to abdominal pain and irregular bowel movement.

Symptoms Of Constipation

Signs of constipation in kids can be abdominal bloating, not passing stool for a few days, passing hard, dry stool, and feeling a loss of appetite. A few other symptoms can also include stool marks on your child's underwear and showing signs of withholding (clenching of teeth, legs crossing, and turning red in the face).

How To Prevent Constipation

Constipation can be prevented by increasing the number of fruits your child eats. Children should eat a healthy amount of fiber to ensure regular bowel movement. They should be discouraged from eating too much junk food and drinking soft drinks as these are high in fat but low in fiber. They should also increase their fluid (especially water) intake.

When To See a Doctor

- Can't function well due to being constipated
- Constipated for longer than 2 weeks
- Has belly pain, fever, or vomiting
- Requires more than the usual amount of pushing to pass stool
- Has small tears on the skin around the anus

Sore Throat

A viral infection, such as the common cold, or environmental conditions, such as dry air, can cause a sore throat. It is more common during the winter or cold seasons, but it can happen at any time of year. It can also be caused by bacterial infections, but this is more likely to result in strep throat. Allergies, as well as smoking, chemicals, and other pollutants, can also cause a sore throat.

Symptoms of a Sore Throat

Pain, itching, or irritation of the throat are all symptoms of a sore throat. Throat pain is the most common symptom of a sore throat. It may get worse as you try to swallow, and you may have trouble swallowing meals and beverages. Your tonsils or throat may appear red at times. Tonsil white patches or pus regions can also occur, but these are more common with strep throat. A sore throat can also cause a runny nose, sneezing, coughing, fever, chills, hoarse voice, headaches, and other symptoms.

How to Prevent Sore Throat

Sore throats, like other common infections, can be avoided by hand washing frequently and not sharing eating utensils or glasses with others. It's also a good idea to stay away from folks who have sore throats or cold symptoms.

When To See a Doctor

Sore throats normally clear up in two to seven days, but they can clear up much faster if you use the natural cures we've suggested.

- Severe sore throat
- Trouble breathing
- Difficulty opening your mouth
- Trouble swallowing
- Sore joints
- A fever higher than 38°C
- Stiff neck
- Earache
- Blood in your saliva or phlegm

If you have a sore throat that lasts more than a week and is accompanied by the above severe symptoms, you should see a doctor.

Nausea

Nausea is described as the uneasiness one feels in the pit of their stomach, and it is usually followed by vomiting. Children can experience nausea because of various reasons, but the most common are gastroenteritis or the stomach flu, food poisoning, or a virus that irritates the gastrointestinal tract.

Symptoms Of Nausea

Signs of nausea can include headache, fever, diarrhea, and even vomiting. Nausea often leads to feeling dizzy, getting headaches, losing appetite, and even abdominal pain.

How To Prevent Nausea

The prevention of nausea highly depends on its cause. However, you can generally prevent nausea by drinking lots of water every day. If your child is prone to nausea but you are sure that they don't have the stomach flu or food poisoning, you can teach them to take deep breaths to help them relax and get rid of the nauseating feeling. You can also give your child some mint tea or lemonade.

When To See a Doctor

Ear Pain

Ear pain or ear aches are sharp pains in one's ears. Teething, sore throat, ear infection, and blocked Eustachian tubes are all possible causes of ear pain. There are two types of them. Acute Otitis Media is the first kind (AOM) and it indicates that fluid behind the eardrum is acutely contaminated. Otitis Media with Effusion is the second kind (OME) and it indicates that there is non-infected fluid in the middle ear. Both are frequently linked to viral upper respiratory infections and are most common in the fall, winter, and spring.

Symptoms of Ear Pain

The most common symptoms of AOM in children include ear pain, fever, irritability, poor sleep, hearing loss, and intermittent ear discharge. This normally goes away on its own in 2 or 3 days, but it can take longer in some cases. On the other hand, hearing loss, with or without ear pain, is one of the most common symptoms of OME. However, it can exist without causing any noticeable symptoms. As long as there is no ear pain or hearing loss that interferes with daily activities, OME will normally go away on its own.

How to Prevent Ear Pain

While many ear infections cannot be infected, there are some steps you can take to reduce your child's risk of developing one. This includes keeping your child away from secondhand smoking, keeping your child in a clean and healthy environment, and breastfeeding your baby for six to twelve months to ensure that they have the antibodies they need to fight infections. Ear Pain in children can also be avoided by properly positioning their bottle so that the formula does not run back into the eustachian tubes, as well as keeping up with their vaccines.

When To See a Doctor

- Ear pain worsens
- Swelling and redness behind the ear
- Ear begins to poke out from the side of the head
- Ear drains pus-like fluid or blood

While most earaches will go away on their own, if your kid is experiencing any serious symptoms, you should call your doctor right away.

Allergies

Allergies are mostly because of one's immune system reacting to a foreign substance that has entered the body. This foreign substance can be pollen, dust, bee venom, pet dander, or even a specific type of food. Children can easily develop allergies, especially if they come from a family with a long history of a particular allergy. They can come in the form of skin rashes, asthma, runny nose, itchy eyes, and an upset stomach. Peanuts and milk are two of the most common allergies for children, so it is best to stay vigilant when feeding these to your children. Each child is different, so a parent should always be aware of their child's allergy and should learn about anaphylaxis – which is a severe, life-threatening allergic reaction that inhibits someone from breathing.

Symptoms Of Allergies

Allergies in children are usually accompanied by itchy, watery eyes and a stuffy or runny nose. Itchiness of ears and roof of the mouth can also be experienced. Their skin may also appear red and dry, and hives or rashes can also appear. Children with asthma can have trouble breathing, coughing, and wheezing. In the most severe cases, children can experience anaphylaxis which causes shortness of breath, vomiting, diarrhea, fainting, and even death.

How To Prevent Allergies

Allergies can be experienced by any child, especially if someone from their family is already experiencing allergies. These can happen and appear at any age, so it's best to remain vigilant about what your child is eating and the environment they are in often. In case your child is allergic to something in their environment (like pollen), it is best to let them play indoors or outdoors only when it isn't the pollen season. In case your child is allergic to a specific type of food, you can prevent them from having allergic reactions by taking that food out of your family's diet, or using dedicated frying pans, cutting boards, utensils, etc.

When To See a Doctor

When your child has been experiencing an allergic reaction for more than a week, even after using over-the-counter drugs or natural remedies, it is best to seek help from a doctor immediately.

Skin Infection

A skin infection occurs when bacteria or other germs penetrate the skin through a wound and spread throughout the body, resulting in pain, swelling, and discoloration. It's a common childhood ailment that can affect any part of the body, including the mouth. Bacteria such as staph and strep are the most common causes. Germs such as viruses, fungi, and parasites can also cause it. Eczema, which causes cracks in the skin and allows bacteria to enter, might raise a child's risk of skin infection. Chickenpox, scrapes, insect bites, animal bites, and puncture wounds are some of the other causes.

Symptoms of Skin Infections

Skin infections come in a variety of forms. Bacterial, fungal, viral, and yeast skin infections are among them. Erythema Multiforme, which can be bacterial, fungal, viral, or yeast in nature, is also included. The signs and symptoms of skin infections vary depending on the type of infection. Red, itchy skin, rashes, inflammation and swelling, fever, painful rashes, and raised bumps are some of the symptoms.

How to Prevent Skin Infections

In any setting, hygiene is critical to preventing the spread of skin infections. You should instruct your youngsters to thoroughly wash their hands with soap and scour all surfaces. To avoid dangerous skin infections, any scratches, scrapes, or rashes caused by allergic reactions should be kept clean and covered. If a member of the household has a skin illness, no one should share towels, linens, or clothing until the infection is completely treated.

When To See a Doctor

If you see that the skin illness is spreading from one family member to another, you should contact your doctor right away so that it may be properly treated. If your kid has a major wound that may be infected, or if your child becomes feverish or unwell because of the wound, you should call your doctor.

Common Cold

The common cold is a viral infection that affects one's nose and throat. It is usually harmless but rhinoviruses, which are the most usual causes of the common cold, can trigger asthma attacks. Children are prone to getting colds during the winter season, but they can also catch it when they attend school or daycare especially if someone there has it. The common cold is a virus, meaning it can't be treated with antibiotics.

Symptoms Of Common Cold

Your child may have a common cold if they have a blocked/stuffy or runny nose and a sore throat. If so, it is possible that they are also experiencing a headache, fever (raised temperature), and a cough.

How To Prevent Common Cold

Children often get colds from the people around them. These can be their teacher or classmates at their daycare, their babysitter, and even their immediate family members. The best way to prevent this is by telling them to constantly wash their hands, avoid touching their face (eyes and mouth) often, and distance themselves from people who have colds.

When To See a Doctor

- Raised temperature or fever for more than 2 days
- Trouble breathing which leads to wheezing
- Earache
- Lack of appetite
- Severe throat pain or cough

Common colds are, like the name implies, common, so medication isn't exactly necessary to treat them. However, if the cold persists for three weeks or more, or if they go away and come back again, you should go see a doctor.

Cough

A cough is the human body's way of removing irritants. It can be voluntary or involuntary, and it is an act that clears one's throat and breathing passage. Coughs aren't considered as a sign of a serious condition most of the time it helps protect and clear the airways in the throat and chest.

Symptoms Of Cough

There are many different types of coughs. For children, the most common are dry and wet coughs. Dry coughs can come from a simple cold or even an inhaled object. Wet coughs are usually accompanied by mucus or phlegm. Various viral infections, like the common cold, influenza, pneumonia, and bronchiolitis, can also cause coughing, so it is important to be sure of the reason why your child is coughing.

How To Prevent Cough

Most coughs, like the common cold, don't really require any immediate medical attention. You don't have to buy cough medicines unless your doctor prescribes one for your child. Coughs are viruses, which run their course for two weeks. However, if your child's cough doesn't stop or persist for more than that, then it may be best to see a doctor.

When To See a Doctor

- Trouble breathing or talking
- Wheezing
- Vomiting
- Drooling or can't swallow well
- Chest pain when inhaling deeply
- Coughing blood
- Has a fever of over 104 degrees Fahrenheit or 40 degrees Celsius with no signs of improvement even after being given fever medicine

Pain

Back pain, stomach pain, head pain, and a range of other painful diseases can affect children. In children and adolescents, chronic or recurrent pain is prevalent. Headaches, abdominal discomfort, chest pain, and limb pain are among them. According to studies, up to 30% to 40% of people experience pain at least once a week.

Abdominal Pain

Viral infections or something more serious, such as appendicitis, can cause abdominal pain. Cramping, diarrhea, gas, bloating, nausea, and vomiting are some of the symptoms that can occur depending on the origin of the pain.

Headaches

Headaches are frequently linked to viral infections. Migraines, tension headaches, cluster headaches, and chronic daily headaches are examples of diverse types of headaches. Migraines can include pulsing or throbbing head pain, a discomfort that gets worse with movement, nausea, vomiting, abdominal pain, and excessive light and sound sensitivity. Tension headaches are characterized by a pressing tightness in the head or neck muscles, mild to severe pain on the sides of the head, and discomfort that is exacerbated by physical activity. Cluster headaches are uncommon in children under the age of ten, although they typically occur in groups of five or more episodes, ranging from one every other day to eight every day. It can also cause teary eyes, congestion, a runny nose, restlessness, or agitation on one side of the head. Finally, an illness or a small head injury might produce chronic daily headaches (CDH). Migraines and tension-type headaches that last more than 15 days per month are frequently included.

Symptoms of Pain

Often, signs of pain in children include reluctance in doing any type of physical activity, irritability, crankiness, lack of appetite, change in sleep schedules, and even non-verbal communication cues like frowning, wincing, or gasping. The symptoms of the many types of pain that children feel are all distinct. It's critical to keep a watch on these symptoms because if left ignored, they can lead to more serious problems.

How to Prevent Pain

The type of pain depends on your child. If it is something caused by a physical injury, prevent this from happening again by teaching or telling your child to be more cautious. You can also reduce the amount of time they spend doing the activity that caused them pain. If it is from growing pains, you can ease what they're feeling using pain relief medication or even natural remedies. If it is from a headache, stomachache, or leg pain, you can wait and see if the pain comes and goes. If it persists, determine the reason why your child is experiencing this. Often, but not always, stress is the number one reason why children feel pain.

When To See a Doctor

- For abdominal pain (stomachache), if it lasts 1 week or longer
- If the pain does not improve or becomes more severe even after giving the child medication or remedy

- Nausea or vomiting due to pain
- Fever higher than 104 degrees Fahrenheit or 40 degrees Celsius

It is not easy to determine whether or not your child is truly in pain. However, if you can see that it is truly affecting their daily life or experiencing the aforementioned severe symptoms, it is best to seek medical advice immediately.

CHAPTER FOUR: RECIPES OF HERBAL REMEDIES FOR CHILDREN

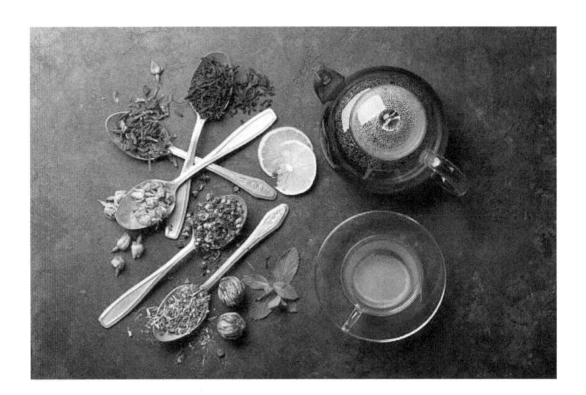

Chamomile

Homemade Chamomile Cough Syrup

The ingredients used in this homemade cough syrup have a long history of being wonderful, effective healers of coughs and colds. They are affordable and easy to get; chances are, you already have most of them in your kitchen right now! You can give your child one tablespoon of this remedy to make them feel better.

Ingredients:

1 tablespoon dried chamomile

6 fresh sage leaves or ½ tablespoon dried sage

Ginger, thinly sliced or grated

1 cup water

½ -¾ cup raw honey

Cinnamon stick for taste

Directions:

1. Add 1 cup of water and the ginger and cinnamon stick to a small saucepan.
2. Simmer on medium-low for 15-20 minutes until the water has reduced by half.
3. Once the water and ginger have reduced, bring the water to a low boil, then turn off the pot and add the sage and chamomile. Cover the pot for 5-10 minutes to steep.
4. Strain the ginger, chamomile, and sage into a jar with a seal of choice.
5. Once the liquid is cooled, add in your honey, and seal the jar.

Chamomile Cough Drops

This is a great remedy for youngsters with colds. All you need are a few items like silicone molds and a candy thermometer to make homemade cough drops that can ease your children's symptoms and make them feel better.

Ingredients:

1½ cups honey

1 cup strong herbal tea

4-6 drops lemon essential oil

Candy Thermometer

Silicone Candy Molds

Directions:

1. Put two tea bags into one cup of water in a saucepan.
2. Heat the water and tea bags to a simmer on high heat. Cover and reduce the heat. Steep for 15 to 20 minutes over the lowest heat.
3. Save ½ cup of the tea for cough drops.
4. Put the herbal tea into a saucepan, then add the honey.
5. Use medium to medium-high heat to heat the ingredients. Keep stirring constantly so that all the ingredients are mixed.
6. Monitor the temperature with a thermometer. You will want it to get to about 300 degrees Fahrenheit.
7. The mixture may get foamy as it heats up. If this occurs, stir.
8. Once the mixture gets near the correct temperature, it will get much thicker. This should take about 30 minutes.
9. Once the liquid reaches 300 degrees Fahrenheit, remove it from the heat.
10. Next, add your essential oils and stir.
11. Transfer the mixture into a Pyrex measuring cup so you can pour it into your silicone molds.
12. Pour very carefully.

13. Allow the cough drops to harden and cool in the candy molds before you store them.

14. Once they have cooled, take the cough drops out of the molds. You can then coat them with powdered stevia, erythritol, or powdered sugar.

15. Store them in single layers between wax paper in the refrigerator for about 3 weeks.

Chamomile Herb Tea

Teas made from chamomile flowers are great for drinking after dinner and before bedtime. It can help your child relax because of its calming and soothing properties. This chamomile herb tea can aid in digestion and lessen the symptoms of coughs and colds.

Ingredients:

2 tablespoons fresh chamomile flowers

2 cups boiling water

2 slices apples (thin slices)

Honey

Directions:

1. Rinse the chamomile flowers with cool water.
2. Warm your teapot with boiling water.
3. Add the apple slices to the pot and mash them using a wooden spoon.
4. Add the chamomile flowers and pour in the boiling water from your teapot.
5. Cover and steep for 3-5 minutes.
6. Strain the tea into two cups.
7. Add honey to taste.
8. Serve hot or cold.

Chamomile Lotion

The therapeutic effects of chamomile are well-known. It has antibacterial and anti-inflammatory characteristics that can help your youngster feel better. It relieves pain by relaxing sore muscles and alleviating any discomfort your child may be experiencing.

Ingredients for Chamomile-Infused Oil:

1 cup dried chamomile flowers

½ cup sweet almond oil

Ingredients for chamomile lotion:

90g distilled water

11g emulsifying wax

25g chamomile-infused oil

2g geogard ultra

5 drops of chamomile essential oil (optional)

Directions:

1. Begin preparing the chamomile-infused oil two weeks before making the lotion. Fill a container halfway with sweet almond oil and a cup of dried chamomile flowers. Place the jar in a cupboard after sealing it.

2. Strain the chamomile-infused oil through a strainer after two or more weeks.

3. In a heat-proof glass jar, combine the emulsifying wax and infused oil, and in another, combine the distilled water. In a large pot, combine both jars. Fill the pan halfway with boiling water.

4. Bring to a boil, then lower to low heat and keep warm. Heat for at least 20 minutes, or until the contents of the jar reach 75 degrees Celsius.

5. Into the oil mixture, pour the distilled water. It should turn a milky opaque tint. Allow cooling after gently stirring for a few minutes. After five minutes, return for another stir.

6. The mixture will thicken to a light lotion consistency as it cools. Return to gently stir every twenty minutes or so.

7. To act as a preservative, add the geogard ultra. You can also use chamomile essential oil, but it's not required.

8. Transfer the lotion to a container and close it. You can use it right away or save it for later.

Ginger

Ginger Honey Lemon Tonic

This tonic is perfect for when your youngster has the flu, an upset stomach, or a sore throat. It's also great for chilly winter days. This tonic is very soothing and healing, and it can be taken in advance when you or your child feel like you're about to come down with something.

Ingredients:

1 cup water

1 piece of 1-inch fresh ginger (or more depending on taste), peeled and chopped

½ medium lemon

1 teaspoon honey

Directions:

1. Place the water, ginger, lemon juice, and honey in a small saucepan over medium heat until heated through.
2. Pour the mixture through a strainer into a mug.

Ginger Milk

For many years, ginger has been used to treat nausea and stomach issues. It relieves stomach ache pain and has several other health benefits. It's an anti-inflammatory that can help with a variety of stomach problems. This dish is great for youngsters, and it can be administered before bedtime to get the best results.

Ingredients:

1 cup milk

1 tablespoon palm sugar

¼ teaspoon dry ginger powder

¼ teaspoon black pepper powder

Directions:

1. In a saucepan, heat 1 cup of milk until it is foamy. When the water has to a boil, add the palm sugar and ginger powder.
2. Mix thoroughly for 2 to 3 minutes. Serve the milk after straining it.

Ginger Cough Syrup

This is a homemade cough syrup made of ginger and a few other ingredients. It's great for sore throats and coughs. It will greatly soothe your youngster's tickly, itchy throat and allow them to be comfortable enough to rest and sleep. Adults are advised to take 2-3 spoonfuls every few hours or as needed, so you should determine the recommended dosage for your child.

Ingredients:

1 teaspoon fresh grated ginger OR ¼ teaspoon ground ginger

¼ teaspoon cayenne pepper

1 clove garlic, grated (optional)

2 tablespoons raw honey

1 tablespoon apple cider vinegar

2 tablespoons water (optional)

<u>*Directions:*</u>

1. Place all ingredients in a small jar with a tight lid.
2. Shake to combine or whisk vigorously in a medium bowl.

Herbal Ginger Brew

This is a great brew for stomach cramps, indigestion, and nausea. It is an energy stimulant and can be used to cure sore throat and coughs.

<u>*Ingredients:*</u>

Syrup

½ cup peeled sliced ginger

1 cup water

¼ cup pure maple syrup

1 cup carbonated water

1 tablespoon lemon juice

Grated lemon, rind

<u>*Directions:*</u>

1. For syrup combine water and ginger in a saucepan, simmer for 30 minutes.
2. Cool slightly and strain.
3. Add maple syrup, stir to mix.
4. Stir 2 tablespoons of syrup into carbonated water, add lemon juice, and peel.

Herbal Blends

Immune Booster Herbal Blend

This herbal blend is perfect for youngsters feeling attacked by the flu season. It boosts their immunity, treats the symptoms of colds and cases of flu, and eases sore throats. This remedy has a pleasant berry flavor that will surely appeal to your child's delicate palate. Adults can drink this herbal blend 1-3 times a day when they feel the telltale signs of a coming cold, so you can base off of that and give your child the necessary dosage. At least once or so a day should be good enough.

<u>*Ingredients:*</u>

4 tablespoons dried elderberries

4 tablespoons dried rose hips

4 tablespoons echinacea root

4 tablespoons astragalus

4 tablespoons dried ginger

Directions:

1. Combine all herbs in a small jar. Stir until evenly distributed.
2. Combine 1-2 tablespoons herbal tea blend per 1-cup water in a small pot.
3. Simmer for 30 minutes.
4. Strain and enjoy hot or iced.

Sleep Aid Herbal Blend

This natural mix of herbs is great for youngsters with insomnia. It also improves their mood and overall outlook. Adults are recommended to take ½ teaspoon a day, so you can adjust the dosage for your child. Do keep in mind that most herbs should not be taken continuously. It is recommended to take this blend two weeks on and one week off or only when needed.

Ingredients:

1 St. John's wort herb, powder

1 valerian root, powder

Directions:

1. Mix herbs together and consume by mixing with juice, food, or putting in an empty capsule.

Delightful Herbal Blend

This wonderful herbal blend can be used not only as a calming, feel-good drink but also as a tea party drink. It is absolutely safe for kids, and adding milk and honey is a great way to enhance the flavor.

Ingredients:

1 teaspoon Spearmint

1 teaspoon Hibiscus

1 teaspoon Chamomile or Lavender

1 teaspoon Sage

1 teaspoon Lemon Peel

Milk or Honey to taste

Directions:

1. Combine herbs in a tea strainer, bag, or infuser.
2. Pour 2-4 cups of boiling water.
3. Let steep for approximately 3-5 minutes.
4. Allow to cool and add milk or honey to taste.

Great Taste Tea Blend

This herbal tea blend not only tastes great, but it also smells great too! It's perfect for kids who are picky about what they drink. It also includes peppermint, which is a great herb that kids recognize and is considered children's favorite.

Ingredients:

1 teaspoon Lemon Balm

1 teaspoon Peppermint

1 teaspoon Oatstraw

1 teaspoon Lycii (Goji) Berries

1 teaspoon Red Clover

Directions:

1. Combine herbs in a tea infuser, bag, or tea nest and pour 3-4 cups boiling water over.
2. Let steep for 3-5 minutes and enjoy.
3. Add a little lemon, milk, or honey.

Turmeric

Fresh Turmeric Tonic

Turmeric is great for you and your child's health. Research has led us to believe that turmeric has the ability to destroy cancer cells, regulate insulin, detox the liver, and clear the skin. This tonic is nourishing and flavorful but be careful with the amount of turmeric you use as it has a very strong flavor which your child may not be accustomed to.

Ingredients:

4 medium organic carrots (4 cups)

1 small golden beet (optional) 2- 3 inches in diameter, cut in half

1 orange (peeled)

1–2 tablespoons sliced fresh turmeric root (start conservatively), peels are okay

1–2 tablespoons fresh ginger

1 apple, cored and quartered

Directions:

1. Juice all ingredients through a juicer.
2. Serve chilled.

Turmeric Milk for Toddlers and Kids

Turmeric is quite unpopular with youngsters because of its strong, almost-peppery flavor. However, it possesses healing abilities that are sure to be beneficial to you and your family. This recipe can be given to kids with coughs and colds. The addition of milk and sugar is sure to mask the turmeric's overwhelming taste, and this may even become your kid's favorite drink!

Ingredients:

1 ½ cups Milk

⅛ teaspoon Turmeric powder

¼ teaspoon Pepper powder

2 tablespoons Palm sugar

Directions:

1. Put the milk in a saucepan and add turmeric powder, palm sugar, and the pepper powder to it and then mix well.
2. Heat the milk under low heat until it is frothy.
3. Pour it into glasses and enjoy.

Cozy Golden Milk

A golden milk is usually made of 2 things: turmeric and coconut (or any other non-dairy-based) milk. This special golden milk is best to drink before going to bed. It is sure to give your youngster a warm, cozy feeling that will ensure sweet dreams.

Ingredients:

2 cups vanilla-flavored coconut milk no sugar added

1 tablespoon turmeric freshly grated

½ tablespoon ginger freshly grated

½ teaspoon cinnamon

⅛ teaspoon nutmeg

1 tablespoon honey

1 pinch black pepper

Directions:

1. Heat everything in a saucepan over medium-low heat. Whisk a you heat it until warmed through and then remove from heat.
2. Pour the mixture through a strainer to remove grated pieces of ginger and turmeric.
3. Pour into mugs.
4. If you wish, garnish it with a cinnamon stick and a sprinkle of nutmeg.

Turmeric Vitamin C Shots with Honey

This tasty turmeric drink includes orange juice, ginger, and honey – some of the best ingredients used to defeat colds and cases of flu. It can easily be done using simple kitchen ingredients, and it is easier to give to your children than the usual vitamin C supplements.

Ingredients:

½ cup 100% Florida Orange Juice

1 teaspoon fresh turmeric, grated

¼ teaspoon fresh ginger, grated

Pinch black pepper

1 teaspoon honey

1 tablespoon hot water

Directions:

1. In a heat-proof glass, add turmeric, ginger, pepper, and honey.
2. Pour hot water into the glass and stir to dissolve honey.
3. Add orange juice and stir to combine.

Turmeric Paste

Turmeric's therapeutic qualities have long been known. It possesses antibacterial, antifungal, and antiviral characteristics that can aid youngsters with skin infections. In addition, the recipe contains coconut oil, which helps to prevent viral or bacterial skin infections, as well as yogurt, which is high in probiotics that are beneficial to your skin.

NATURAL REMEDIES FOR CHILDREN

Ingredients:

¼ teaspoon organic turmeric powder

1 tablespoon extra-virgin coconut oil

1 tablespoon Greek yogurt

Water

Directions:

1. Organic turmeric powder should be heated in water over extremely low heat for around six to eight minutes, stirring constantly.

2. Stir in the remaining ingredients – coconut oil and Greek yogurt – once the rice has been cooked and formed into a thick paste.

3. Continue to whisk until the coconut oil has completely melted. Allow time for cooling.

4. Refrigerate for up to three weeks after transferring to a glass container.

Herbal Ointments, Salves, and Rubs

Herbal Anti-Inflammatory Ointment

This anti-inflammatory ointment can be used as a chest rub for colds. It soothes the inflammation caused by coughing. The plantains mentioned in this recipe are little green plants growing as weeds in various places, not green bananas.

Ingredients:

1 cup fresh plantain, plants

½ cup oil

Directions:

1. Wash and coarsely chop plantain. You can use the whole plant or just the leaves.

2. Mix with oil in the saucepan and heat to boiling.

3. Turn off the burner and allow plants to sit in the oil until it has cooled completely.

4. Strain oil and discard plants.

5. Store in an airtight container.

6. Apply externally to inflamed areas.

Herbal Rub for Bruises and Inflammation

This herbal rub is used to dissolve bruises and lessen pain caused by inflammation (muscle pains). It takes only a bit of time to prepare, and it provides temporary relief which your child will surely be grateful for.

Ingredients:

½ cup arnica dried fresh edible flower, whole

½ cup St. John's wort flowers, cut

1 teaspoon cayenne pepper, powder

¼ - ½ cup olive oil

Directions:

1. In a saucepan, heat or slowly simmer equal parts of the premixed herbs with olive oil or lard for several hours or longer.
2. Allow to cool.
3. Strain and bottle the oil for use as needed.

Homemade Salve for Eczema

This homemade salve is great for soothing dry skin and itchy skin caused by eczema. It is made of healing ingredients, mostly consisting of essential oils that soothe both the appearance of your youngster's skin as well as the itchiness they are feeling. It helps reduce the symptoms of the rash and lessens its amount, but if the rash comes back, you should consider taking your child to a doctor for a check-up.

Ingredients:

½ cup shea butter

½ cup coconut oil

¼ cup beeswax

1 tablespoon raw honey

10 drops lavender essential oil

8 drops frankincense

5 drops Tea Tree essential oil

5 drops geranium essential oil

Directions:

1. Melt shea butter, coconut oil, and beeswax in a double boiler.
2. Let mixture cool slightly.
3. Add raw honey and essential oils.

4. Mix well and pour into a shallow tin.

5. Allow it to harden before applying to the area of concern.

Herbal Salve for Headaches

This herbal salve can be used when your youngster feels bad and complains about having a headache. Headaches can be caused by many things, and, unfortunately, even children can experience them. We all know how irritating and tiring it feels to battle a headache. This salve is applied on the forehead, temples, neck, shoulders, or whichever area needs some cooling tension relief.

Ingredients:

½ oz beeswax

4 Tablespoons extra virgin olive oil

2 Tablespoons castor oil

1 Tablespoon magnesium oil

20 drops peppermint essential oil

10 drops lavender essential oil

10 drops citrus essential oil

Directions:

1. Place beeswax and olive oil in a double boiler to melt. Use a low heat setting to preserve the integrity of the oil.

2. Remove from heat and add the magnesium, castor, and the essential oils. Whip it quickly with a fork and pour into a glass.

3. Place in your refrigerator or freezer to set. Remove when hardened – this should be no more than 30 minutes.

Essential Oils

Tea Tree Oil Ear Drops

This formula for natural ear infection drops contains antibacterial and anti-inflammatory characteristics that can help your child's discomfort and infection. Olive oil contains antibacterial and antiviral characteristics, garlic has various herbal properties and is a common ingredient in home treatment, and tea tree oil has antimicrobial capabilities.

Ingredients:

2 tablespoons olive oil or fractionated coconut oil

2 cloves of crushed garlic

6-8 drops of tea tree oil

Directions:

1. Heat oil in a small pan and add crushed garlic. Cook over low heat until garlic becomes fragrant. It will usually take around 3-4 minutes for the garlic to infuse in the oil. Remove from heat.
2. Strain the oil and pour it into a sterile dropper bottle. Add 6-8 drops of tea tree oil and shake well.
3. Drop 1-2 drops into the ear as needed. Have your child lie on their side and gently massage behind their ears. Wait 5 minutes until the oil has been absorbed by the ear. Use once per day as needed.

Essential Oil Spray

You can use any essential oil you like for this recipe. Symptom alleviation was observed 20 minutes after applying a spray containing eucalyptus citriodora, eucalyptus globulus, peppermint, oregano, and rosemary, according to one study.

Ingredients:

10-20 drops of essential oils of choice

Distilled or filtered water

1 tablespoon grain alcohol (as preservative)

2 oz spray bottle

Directions:

1. Combine 10-20 drops of essential oils with grain alcohol. Fill the bottle with water, add the spray top, and shake vigorously.
2. Before using, give it a good shake.

Sweet Dreams Essential Oil Spray

This is great for using before bedtime. Geranium essential oils have been used to treat anxiety, depression, and manage pain for a long time. Roman chamomile essential oils are sweet, helping to create a calming and relaxing atmosphere for your child that is sure to help them fall asleep.

Ingredients:

2 teaspoons fractionated coconut oil

3 drop Roman Chamomile essential oil

2 drop Geranium essential oil

1 10ml bottle

Directions:

1. Combine the coconut oil and essential oils in the roller bottle.
2. Store away from the reach of young children.

Essential Oil Chest Rub

This chest rub is made of essentially only 2 elements: a balm and essential oils. The balm acts as a carrier when it comes in contact with warm skin, and it allows the essential oils to properly do their job without harming your youngster. Applying this just before bedtime allows your children to fall asleep feeling more relaxed and comfortable.

Ingredients:

4 teaspoons beeswax

7 Tablespoons coconut oil

3 Tablespoons shea butter

10 drops eucalyptus oil

15 drops tea tree oil

5 drops lavender oil

Directions:

1. Take two pots, preferably one that can fit and be put into the other.
2. Add 2 cups of water to the big pot and then put the second smaller pot inside. The smaller pot should not touch the bottom of the bigger one.
3. Bring the water to boil.
4. Add the beeswax to the small pot and let it melt.
5. Add shea butter, melt it, and remove from the heat.
6. Add coconut oil and essential oils and mix well.
7. Pour everything into a glass container or mason jar with a lid.
8. Let it cool and it will transform into a solid cream.

Lavender Essential Oil Salve

This natural, herb-infused semi-solid ointment is great for dry skin, small cuts, bruises, and irritations. It's the perfect thing to apply when your youngster falls off a swing or accidentally scrapes their knee while running. The ingredients used are affordable and absolutely easy to get.

Ingredients:

¾ cup of calendula oil

¼ cup coconut oil

1 oz of beeswax

15-18 drops of lavender essential oil

Pinch of dried turmeric powder

Directions:

1. Using a double boiler, add water to the bottom pot, and then pour calendula oil into the top pot and place above. You can also make your own makeshift double boiler if you don't have one. Just keep in mind that the oil needs non-direct and even heat to prevent burning.
2. Bring your double boiler to low heat and grate in your beeswax, and then add in coconut oil.
3. Once everything has melted, add your lavender essential oil and a large pinch of turmeric powder.
4. Stir the mixture, and then quickly turn off your burner.
5. Slowly and carefully pour the mixture into a tin and allow the salve to cool.

Garlic

Garlic Milk

This remedy can boost your youngster's immunity and treat cold-related symptoms as well as digestive issues. It is not considered a kid-favorite since garlic has an unpleasant taste for some, but it's good for the body. However, garlic can be quite intense for some kids, so you should remember to give garlic milk in moderation.

Ingredients:

1 ½ cups Milk

2 tablespoons Palm Sugar

3 cloves Garlic

Directions:

1. Take garlic cloves and roughly mince them in a mortar and pestle. Set this aside for 5 minutes
2. Boil milk in a saucepan until frothy

3. Lower the flame. Add minced garlic and palm candy.

4. Mix well and boil it further for 5 mins on low flame

5. Once the garlic is soft, switch off the flame and serve the milk warm

Garlic Oil Ointment

This remedy is used to get rid of sniffles, coughs, and touches of the flu. It is an ointment and a rub, so it directly transfers garlic's antibacterial, antiviral, and antifungal properties from your skin and into your bloodstream. This ointment is best rubbed on the chest and feet, which are then covered with socks.

Ingredients:

¼ Cup Coconut Oil
6 Peeled Garlic Cloves

Directions:

1. Process all ingredients in a food processor. Melt your coconut oil on the stove over low heat slightly if needed. Process until a smooth salve/ointment.

2. Store in a glass jar.

3. Store in the fridge for up to 6 months. Let it come to room temperature when you need to use it.

Garlic Salve for Coughs and Colds

Garlic has been known to have incredible healing properties, so this nice, smelly, homemade salve can be used to lessen your child's cough, cold, and fever. You can rub it onto your child's chest or on the soles of their feet and repeat every 2-3 hours until their condition improves.

Ingredients:

8 cloves garlic, peeled
⅓ cup coconut oil
10 drops lavender oil

Directions:

1. Combine the ingredients together in a food processor or blender.

2. Blend for about 3 minutes, or until it is a perfectly smooth whipped butter of sorts. You may need to scrape the sides of the food processor to get all the garlic into the paste.

3. Put into a small container and refrigerate.

Fermented Garlic Honey

Garlic has a very strong aroma and equally intense taste that makes children veer off of it. However, it is one of the most potent ingredients that easily fights off touches of flu and colds. This fermented remedy can be used at any given moment that your child seems to be coming down with something. You can use a syringe and administer 1ml to your kid and it will fight off any signs of cold straight away.

Ingredients:

1 bulb organic, local garlic

1 cup local raw honey (enough to cover cloves)

Directions:

1. Peel and smash the cloves of garlic with the side of your knife.
2. Place into a sterilized jam jar and pour in enough honey to cover it. The jar should be large enough to allow the contents to double in size. Close tightly with the lid.
3. Wait for 2-4 weeks for it to ferment.
4. You need to open the jar to release excess carbon dioxide once a day and flip it upside down to ensure all the cloves are constantly coated in honey.
5. Fermentation begins once bubbles start forming. If this hasn't started within 4 days, add 1 teaspoon of water and continue the steps above.
6. Continue doing this until the bubbles stop, the honey is thin, and the cloves have sunk to the bottom. This could be a month or more.
7. Store in the fridge and it will continue to age. It will last for years if stored in a dark spot.

CONCLUSION

Herbal remedies have been around for thousands of years. They are now widely used by people in the United States. They are, however, not for everyone. Herbal remedies are contentious since they are not subject to scrutiny by the FDA or other regulatory authorities. The evidence for the efficacy of herbal medications is often lacking. Although some people find them useful, their use is frequently based on tradition rather than scientific evidence.

According to a new study, herbal medicines appear to be more helpful in children than in adults. This does not, however, imply that it is inherently safer. According to Contemporary Pediatrics, roughly 12% of families give their children herbs and vitamins, and that proportion jumps to nearly 50% for children with chronic illnesses. Natural items including fish oil, melatonin, and probiotics were the most popular herbs and supplements among youngsters. Back or neck discomfort, other musculoskeletal disorders, head or chest colds, anxiety or stress, attention-deficit hyperactivity disorder (ADHD), and insomnia or trouble sleeping were the most common uses. Before you consider utilizing herbal medicines to treat your child's sickness, make sure you conduct some research and consult with your doctor to ensure that it is safe.

Because there are so many alternatives when it comes to using natural medicines, it is critical that you conduct thorough research to determine what is and is not safe for your children. Gingko, echinacea, peppermint, arnica, chamomile, turmeric, and ginger are some of the herbs and spices that are considered safe for children. Other substances like belladonna and ephedra, on the other hand, should be avoided. While researching every plant or spice you come across may be time-consuming, it is the only way to verify that anything you are using to treat your child will not cause extra harm. Along with ensuring that the herbs and spices you're using are safe, always double-check that you're utilizing the right one for your purposes. If you're looking for a way to help your youngster with a sore throat, ginger is a good choice. You don't want to utilize anything that will aggravate your child's symptoms.

While some herbs and spices are acceptable for children, you should still be cautious about the amount you give them. Although an herb or spice may be healthy, giving your child too much of it could be harmful. The organs of your children are smaller and more vulnerable to harm. You should carefully regulate the dosage you give your children, just as you would with traditional medicine, and follow your doctor's or specialist's recommendations. This book contains a chapter that allows you to learn about the recommended dosage of tea, tincture, etc. for your child, however, if you are still skeptical or unsure about how much of a certain remedy you should give your child, you can always drop by a professional's office and ask them.

If you wish to give your children herbal treatments, make sure to read the labels carefully and only use the recommended dosage. Never take more than the stated dosage and find out who should not use the supplement. Reduce the dosage or stop using the herbal supplement if symptoms such as nausea, dizziness, headache, or upset stomach occur. Be on the lookout for any allergic reactions. You should always conduct a patch test first before using any herb on your child. This can be done by taking a small sample of whatever herb or spice you plan to use and applying it on your child's skin, particularly and preferably on their arm. If your child experiences any negative reactions or you see that they are having problems breathing, or if another problem arises, call your local emergency number for assistance right away.

Your children are treated with herbal remedies, not cured. They may help to lessen pain and symptoms, but they will not be able to entirely treat your child. Your child will still need to see a doctor, particularly if they are experiencing severe symptoms. Your doctor may still prescribe pharmaceuticals that are more effective than natural therapies, but if you choose to utilize herbal medicine, always seek medical advice first. It's critical that you understand this, so you don't have unrealistic hopes for a certain herb or spice and are disappointed when your child isn't cured by the end of the week.

If you wish to utilize natural remedies to treat a specific condition, see your doctor first to ensure that they will not interact with any medications your child is taking. It's essential that your doctor understands your child's worries and why you want to use the treatments in the first place. If you're concerned about your child's growth or appetite, for example, consult your doctor first to be sure there isn't something more serious going on. While doctors may not be well-versed in alternative therapies, they nevertheless care about your child's well-being and will want to ensure that he or she is healthy.

This book contains not only information on how safe herbal remedies really are for children, but it also includes recipes using herbs and spices that are well-known and popular among herbalists for being effective. Herbs like chamomile, sage, St. John's wort, and hibiscus are part of the key ingredients of most of these recipes. We kept in mind that children are particularly difficult to give and administer medicine to, so we used recipes that can be made tasty using sugar, milk, and honey but are nevertheless still efficient and capable of curing minor illnesses. Spices like turmeric, black pepper, and cayenne pepper were also used. These are only a few of the many spices that are best known for curing symptoms of colds, coughs, and cases of flu.

Many of these natural, herbal treatments are becoming increasingly popular. They've been used by more than one in ten US children, and more than half of US children with chronic medical issues. As the popularity of these therapies grows, spurred in part by what people read on the Internet and social media, it's important that people become informed and educated about them, particularly if they plan to use them on their children.

BOOK 6
NATURAL REMEDIES
FOR ELDERS

CHAPTER ONE: ARE NATURAL REMEDIES SAFE FOR ELDERS?

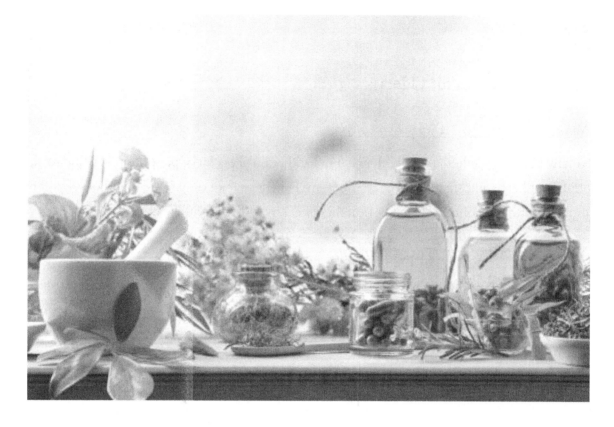

The WHO has estimated that 80 percent of the world's population uses traditional therapies, most of which are derived from plants. In the U.S. alone, one in five people uses herbal products. According to the CDC's National Health Statistics Report, 41% of adults in the United States aged 60 to 69 utilize alternative medicines, including herbal therapy. In a 2002 National Health Interview Survey, it was discovered that half of the respondents polled did not tell conventional doctors about their herb use. Teas, tablets, capsules, liquid extracts (tinctures), powders, and the original roots, leaves, seeds, and flowers are all available in a variety of forms. To enhance health and wellness, a diet can also include a variety of herbs and spices. Of course, certain herbals have been thoroughly examined and proven to be effective for their intended use. Many are also fairly safe, but the term "natural" does not indicate which are safe and which are not.

Some herbs contain strong components that should be treated with the same caution as prescription drugs. In truth, many pharmaceutical drugs are produced from man-made analogs of naturally occurring plant components.

You should first educate yourself about the benefits and drawbacks of natural medicines before deciding to use them. Some natural cures may have unintended consequences, so it's best to do your homework first.

Pros and Cons of Natural Remedies for Elders

Some herbs contain strong components that should be treated with the same caution as prescription drugs. In truth, many pharmaceutical drugs are produced from man-made analogs of naturally occurring plant components. You should first educate yourself about the benefits and drawbacks of natural medicines before deciding to use them. Some natural cures may have unintended consequences, so it's best to do your homework first.

Pros of Natural Remedies for Elders

Pro #1: Natural Remedies Are Always Evolving

Although many herbal remedies are more than a thousand years old, a lot of people are still finding the positive effects of different herbs and spices every day. They are being used not only for teas and oils, but they are also being combined with foods that may make something healthy taste more delicious.

Pro #2: Natural Remedies Have Fewer Chemicals

For many years, herbs and spices have been utilized as medicines. Today, they are also employed in certain modern medicine. The best part about herbal medicines is that they don't include any chemicals. Some medicines and treatments contain chemicals that may be more hazardous, which is why some people prefer to use natural products.

Pro #3: Natural Remedies Are Cheaper

The simple truth is that prescription medications are quite expensive. Herbal medicine is often more affordable because the medications come from abundant natural resources. A lower production cost means a price. Herbal remedies also show people how to to prevent illness and promote self-healing naturally.

Pro #4: Natural Remedies Improve Overall Health

Natural medicines come with many significant health benefits. First, natural cures often aim to identify and eradicate illness rather than act as a band-aid for symptoms. This approach is more likely to result in improved health than the use of pharmaceutical drugs. Also, because herbal medicine contains vitamins, antibodies and other health-promoting agents, it increases one's overall health and not just combat illness.

Pro #5: The Use Of Natural Remedies Is A Part Of A Holistic Lifestyle

Individuals can use their knowledge about natural remedies to lead healthier lifestyles and, hopefully, prevent chronic conditions. When taking natural remedies, you will need to keep up to date with the treatments you are taking. This will improve your habits and help you build an overall better lifestyle.

Regardless of what medicine, herbal remedy, or supplement you choose – it is best to discuss with your doctor beforehand. Your doctor will know of your medical history, and therefore, they know what is best for your safety and health. Herbal remedies – while effective, affordable, and natural, still have a lot of properties that could harm your body instead of making it feel better.

Cons of Natural Remedies for Elders

Con #1: Natural Remedies Can Be Unsafe For Some Individuals

There is no telling how a certain herb or spice would react to a certain individual. There is no set result for herbal remedies, and therefore it could be quite harmful to some. Unlike modern medicine that is tested and ensured for safety, you will not be able to get that peace of mind when it comes to herbal remedies.

Con #2: Natural Remedies Are Not FDA-Approved

The Food and Drug Administration (FDA) has not approved many natural therapies, so there is no guarantee that they will be safe or effective. Because they haven't been tested or put through any clinical trials, there's no way of knowing whether a natural treatment would benefit or harm a person.

Con #3: Natural Remedies May Be Harmful When Combined With Other Medication

It is best to consult with your doctor, especially if you are on any medications or have a chronic health condition. Herbal medicines can react poorly when combined with other medications and they can cause a variety of side effects, ranging from moderate to severe. Allergic reactions and rashes, asthma, headaches, nausea, vomiting, and dizziness are some of the side effects of some herbal medicines.

Con #4: Natural Remedies Can Have Active Components That Are Unknown

Active components can be found in herbal remedies. Many herbal remedies' active components are yet unknown. Herbal medicine practitioners believe that the complete plant has a larger effect than its components. Critics claim that the nature of herbal medicine makes administering a precise amount of an active ingredient challenging.

CHAPTER TWO: COMMON ILLNESSES IN ELDERS

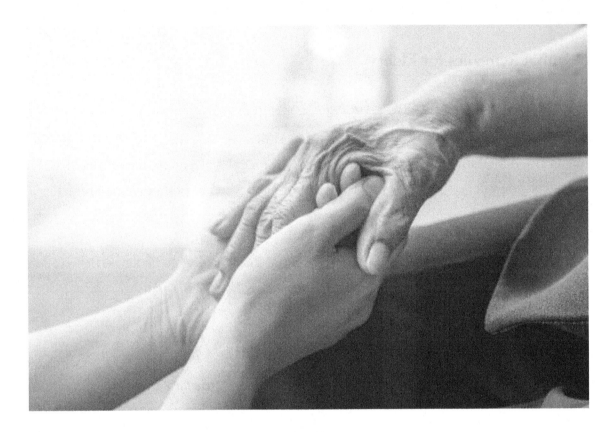

According to the World Health Organization (WHO), more individuals are anticipated to live into their sixties and beyond. This extended life provides chances for older people and their families, as well as for entire societies. These extra years allow these individuals to pursue higher education, begin a new career, or follow a long-neglected hobby. However, one factor is preventing them from reaching their full potential – their health. Aging is caused by the accumulation of a wide range of molecular and cellular damage over time. This can result in a loss of physical and mental capacity, as well as an increased risk of disease and, ultimately, death.

Hearing loss, cataracts, back and neck pain, arthritis, chronic obstructive pulmonary disease, diabetes, depression, and dementia are all frequent illnesses associated with growing older. The older people get, the more likely they are to have many conditions at the same time.

Hearing Loss

Noise, aging, sickness, and genetics are all factors that can lead to hearing loss. Hearing loss affects one out of every three adults between the ages of 65 and 74, and nearly half of those over 75 have difficulties hearing. Because they may not understand what is being said, older persons who can't hear properly may become unhappy, upset, or ashamed. Because of their state, they are incorrectly assumed to be confused, unresponsive, or uncooperative. There are two types of hearing loss: conductive and sensorineural. Conductive hearing loss can easily be treated with a quick and painless procedure. On the other hand, sensorineural hearing loss is significantly more difficult to treat. When there is a problem with the inner ear, specifically the cilia, this form of hearing loss occurs. It is currently incurable, however, it can be treated with hearing aids and cochlear implants, as well as natural medications.

Symptoms of Hearing Loss

Hearing loss can develop slowly over time. The inability to hear high-pitched sounds, difficulty hearing background noises and difficulty hearing people talk are the most common symptoms. Other signs and symptoms include excessively hearing loud sounds, difficulties hearing in noisy environments, ringing in the ears, asking individuals to repeat themselves, turning up the volume on the television or radio more than usual, and more.

Prevention of Hearing Loss

Although age-related hearing loss cannot be prevented, it can be managed to prevent it from worsening. If you have age-related hearing loss, you should limit your exposure to loud noises, use ear protection in noisy environments, and keep your blood sugar under control if you have diabetes. You can also consume meals high in vitamins and minerals including vitamin B12, potassium, and magnesium.

When To See a Doctor

If you detect any of the symptoms of hearing loss, you should contact an audiologist for a comprehensive hearing evaluation. If you are suffering any of the following symptoms, you should get medical advice:

- Sudden onset or rapidly increasing hearing loss
- History of ear discomfort, active discharge, or bleeding
- Visualization of blood, pus, cerumen plug, foreign body, or other material in the ear canal
- Unilateral or asymmetric hearing loss

Cataracts

A cataract is a disorder in which proteins in the lens of the eye break down and clump together, usually owing to aging, physical trauma, or illness. Vision will become hazy as these clumps grow and change; you may experience double vision in one eye; your vision may become yellow or darken, or you may experience haziness similar to fog. Cataracts caused by old age are the most common cause of blindness. Nuclear, cortical, and subcapsular are the three basic forms of cataracts. The most powerful predictor of cataract development is age. Family history of cataracts, diabetes, smoking, obesity, poor nutrition, lower socioeconomic position, and alcohol usage are all risk factors. Surgery is the only way to cure cataracts; all other treatments will just slow the progression of the disease.

Symptoms of Cataracts

Cataracts may appear to be simple cloudiness in your vision at first, and they may only damage a tiny portion of your eyes. However, if the cataract grows larger, it will impair more of your lens. Clouded, blurred, or dim vision, difficulty seeing at night, sensitivity to light and glare, needing a very bright light for reading and other activities, observing halos around lights, requiring frequent changes in eyeglasses or contact lenses, seeing a fading or yellowing of colors, and double vision in one eye are all symptoms of cataracts.

Prevention of Cataracts

Regular eye examinations and a balanced diet, according to several specialists, can help avoid cataracts. You should also avoid smoking and limit alcohol consumption, manage other health issues such as diabetes, and wear sunglasses to protect yourself from ultraviolet B (UVB) rays when outside.

When To See a Doctor

Make an appointment for an eye test right away if you detect any changes in your vision. Double vision or flashes of light are two examples of noticeable alterations in your eyesight. If you have sudden eye pain or headaches, you should consult a doctor right away.

Back and Neck Pain

Back and neck pain is something that all of us experience as we get older. Most people notice back pain between the ages of 40 and 60. The discs in our spine, arthritis, or spinal stenosis are all possible causes of neck and back pain.

Symptoms of Back and Neck Pain

It is estimated that 85 percent of people will suffer from back or neck pain at some point in their lives.

Back Pain

Mornings and evenings are the most prevalent times for back pain. It comprises any combination of pain that keeps you awake at night, a discomfort that gets worse later in the day, localized tenderness when the affected area of the spine is touched, aching, constant, or intermittent pain in the lower back, and back stiffness or lack of flexibility.

Neck Pain

Poor posture or osteoarthritis can cause neck pain, which is a common complaint. Its symptoms include headaches, muscle tightness, and spasms, limited ability to move your head, and pain that is increased by holding your head in one spot for lengthy periods.

Prevention of Back and Neck Pain

The best way to prevent back and neck pain is by improving your posture and modify your seats to ensure you are not slouching in any way. You should also avoid carrying heavy bags and luggage, stretch and stay active, and sleep in a decent position to reduce back and neck problems.

When To See a Doctor

Back and neck discomfort may usually be addressed at home with a little patience. However, if you are suffering any of the following symptoms, you should get medical attention right away:

- Severe pain
- Lasts several days without relief
- Pain spreads down arms or legs
- Is accompanied by a headache, numbness, weakness, or tingling
- Weight loss that isn't explained
- Nighttime pain
- Bladder or bowel incontinence

Arthritis

Arthritis is one of the most prevalent diseases in the United States. This condition affects millions of adults, including half of all people aged 65 and more. Osteoarthritis, rheumatoid arthritis, and gout are common in the elderly. In your joints, cartilage is a tough but flexible connective tissue. It protects your joints by cushioning the pressure and shock that comes with moving and stressing them. Arthritis is caused by a decline in the typical amount of cartilage tissue. Osteoarthritis, one of the most frequent types of arthritis, is caused by normal wear and tear. If you have a family history of OA, your chances of developing it are increased. Rheumatoid Arthritis, another prevalent type of arthritis, is an autoimmune disease. It happens when your immune system targets your body's tissues. The synovium, soft tissue in your joints that creates a fluid that nourishes the cartilage and lubricates the joints, is affected by these attacks. RA is a synovial disease that infiltrates and destroys joints. It can eventually cause both bone and cartilage inside the joint to be destroyed. It's unclear what causes the immune system's attacks. However, scientists have uncovered genetic markers that fivefold enhance your chances of acquiring RA.

Symptoms of Arthritis

Arthritis can strike suddenly or develop gradually over time. Joint pain, stiffness, swelling, tenderness in and around the joint, and heat or redness surrounding the joint are some of the most prevalent symptoms.

Osteoarthritis

Osteoarthritis develops when the body's natural cartilage, which acts as a cushion between two bones, wears off. This is commonly thought to be a byproduct of growing older. As the two bones rub together, the injured cartilage causes pain and suffering. The most common symptoms of osteoarthritis are joint pain and stiffness, which can make it difficult to move the afflicted joints and perform daily tasks.

Rheumatoid Arthritis

Rheumatoid arthritis can strike at any age, and while both men and women are affected, it is more common in women. This type of arthritis is an autoimmune illness in which the body's immune system assaults the joints, causing inflammation and discomfort. Flare-ups can affect any joint in the body, although the neck, shoulders, ankles, knees, hips, elbows, wrists, and fingers are the most commonly affected. It is also symmetrical, affecting both sides of the body at the same time. The heart, neurological system, and blood arteries can all be affected in severe cases of inflammation. Excessive weariness is another symptom of rheumatoid arthritis, which can lead to a fever.

Gout

Gout is a kind of arthritis that happens when uric acid builds up in connective tissue or the spaces between joints. It is one of the most severe types of arthritis. Gout is now known to be triggered by several foods, including anchovies, liver, shrimp, peas, dried beans, and even gravy, and was once thought to be caused solely by ingesting too-rich foods. Being overweight or consuming large amounts of alcohol might also cause gout. The big toe is the most common site of gout, although it can also affect the other toes, as well as the knee, ankle, hand, and wrist.

Prevention of Arthritis

While some types of arthritis are unavoidable, many others can be reduced or slowed by modifying one's lifestyle. Maintaining a healthy weight, avoiding damage to joints, ligaments, and cartilage, and boosting and protecting your immune system are some of the greatest ways to keep joints healthy and prevent degenerative arthritis.

When To See a Doctor

While you can cure arthritis at home, you should visit a doctor if you are suffering any of the following symptoms:

- Multiple painful joints
- Joints that ache a lot
- Pain that doesn't go away with rest
- Joints that turn red or hot
- Pain and stiffness that comes on slowly

Chronic Obstructive Pulmonary Disease (COPD)

COPD, or chronic obstructive pulmonary disease, is extremely frequent in the elderly. It's believed that 10% of Americans aged 75 and over are affected. Even though COPD is extremely widespread, diagnosing older persons with the disease can be difficult. Because aging is accompanied by muscular deconditioning, comorbid diseases, and other factors that contribute to a normal loss in respiratory function - all of which might conceal it. COPD, or chronic obstructive pulmonary disease, is extremely frequent in the elderly. It's believed that 10% of Americans aged 75 and over are affected. Even though COPD is extremely widespread, diagnosing older persons with the disease can be difficult. Because aging is accompanied by muscular deconditioning, comorbid diseases, and other factors that contribute to a normal loss in respiratory function - all of which might conceal it.

Symptoms of Chronic Obstructive Pulmonary Disease

COPD advances at a slower pace. Shortness of breath, a chronic cough, and sputum production are all frequent symptoms among the elderly. They are also unable to maintain normal activities and may have chest tightness and wheezing, as well as a loss of appetite and exhaustion. COPD symptoms in elderly persons can be mistaken for signs of aging. However, it is critical to get them examined.

Prevention of Chronic Obstructive Pulmonary Disease

COPD may not be preventable for everyone, especially when genetics play a role. However, the most effective strategy to avoid COPD is to avoid smoking or to stop smoking if you already do. COPD is most commonly caused by smoking. COPD can be prevented by avoiding contaminants in the airways. Chemicals, secondhand smoke, dust, and fumes are examples of pollutants.

When To See a Doctor

If you are having any of the following severe symptoms, you should see a doctor about COPD:

- Respiratory infections regularly
- Breathlessness
- Fatigue
- Weight loss
- Morning headaches
- Swollen feet and ankles

Diabetes

Diabetes is a dangerous condition that affects a large number of senior citizens. When a person's blood glucose, commonly known as blood sugar, is too high, they get diabetes. The good news is that you can take efforts to avoid or delay type 2 diabetes, which is the most frequent type of diabetes in older people. If you already have diabetes, there are medicines available to help you manage the disease and avoid complications. Type 1 and type 2 diabetes are the two most common types of diabetes. The body does not produce insulin in Type 1 diabetes. Although this type of diabetes can affect older people, it most commonly affects children and young adults, who thereafter develop diabetes for the rest of their lives. The body does not manufacture or utilize insulin as well in Type 2 diabetes. Diabetes mellitus is the most frequent kind of diabetes. It affects middle-aged and older adults the most, but it can also impact youngsters.

Symptoms of Diabetes

If you think you or a loved one might have diabetes, pay attention to these signs and symptoms.

Type 1 Diabetes

Excessive thirst and hunger, frequent urination, unexplained weight loss, and weariness are all symptoms of type 1 diabetes.

Type 2 Diabetes

A person with type 2 diabetes will suffer any of the symptoms that a person with type 1 diabetes would have. They may also have wounds that never heal or heal slowly, as well as confusion, hazy vision, sadness, and numbness or tingling in their feet or hands.

Prevention of Diabetes

Diabetes can be avoided in the elderly by leading a healthy lifestyle. Diabetes can be avoided by eating nutritious and healthy foods and avoiding high-sugar foods, empty carbs, and trans fats. Exercising and restricting alcohol consumption, as well as portion control, stress management, and mental well-being, can all help.

When To See a Doctor

When blood sugar levels become too high, it can lead to more serious problems including entering a coma or even death. If you have any of the following symptoms, contact your doctor right away:

- Gets very tired
- Losing weight
- Extremely hungry
- Always thirsty and pee frequently

Depression

Clinical depression is frequent in the elderly. About 6 million Americans aged 65 and up are affected. However, only 10% of those who are diagnosed obtain therapy. The elderly often have different symptoms of depression than the young. The consequences of various ailments and the medications used to treat them are commonly confused with depression in elderly persons.

Symptoms of Depression

Some elderly persons may not show any signs of depression. Instead, people may be wary, have difficulties sleeping, be cranky or irritated, be confused, struggle to pay attention, lose interest in activities they used to like, move slowly, gain, or lose weight, feel hopeless, worthless, or guilty, suffer from aches and pains, or have suicidal thoughts.

Prevention of Depression

Staying active and socially involved can help prevent depression in the elderly. Exercising is not only healthy for the body, but it can also help with depression, anxiety, and stress. Exercising causes a variety of brain changes, such as neuronal development, reduced inflammation, and new activity patterns that improve sensations of peace and well-being. Furthermore, social isolation is becoming more prevalent among the elderly, which has an impact on their mental and physical health as well as their mortality risk. Being socially engaged can assist to strengthen your immune system, relieve physical pain, and lower blood pressure.

When To See a Doctor

If your symptoms persist for more than two weeks, you should consult a doctor. Frequent symptoms are a clear indication of depression or another health problem. Serious depression can lead to suicide, therefore it's essential not to disregard any warning signals.

Dementia

Dementia is a phrase that refers to a set of symptoms that impact your memory, reasoning, and social abilities to the point where they interfere with your regular activities. Dementia doesn't have just one cause. Memory loss is a common symptom of dementia, but it can be caused by a variety of factors. Memory loss isn't always a marker of dementia but it is usually one of the first symptoms. Alzheimer's disease is the most prevalent cause of progressive dementia in older people, but dementia can also be caused by a variety of other conditions. Some dementia symptoms may be reversible, depending on the reason.

Symptoms of Dementia

Memory loss, difficulty communicating, difficulty with visual and spatial abilities, difficulty reasoning or problem-solving, difficulty handling complex tasks, difficulty planning and organizing, difficulty with coordination and motor functions, as well as confusion and disorientation are all common signs and symptoms of dementia. Personality changes, melancholy, anxiety, inappropriate conduct, paranoia, agitation, and hallucinations are all possible side effects of dementia.

Prevention of Dementia

Although there is no way to avoid dementia, there are strategies to assist in its treatment. Keeping your intellect engaged, as well as being physically and socially active, may be good. It's also a good idea to give up smoking and eat a healthy diet, as well as get enough sleep. Treating any health issues, such as hearing loss or cardiovascular difficulties, can also help minimize the risk of dementia.

When To See a Doctor

If you or a loved one has been suffering memory issues or other dementia symptoms, it is best to see a doctor. This is to establish your true situation, as various medical diseases might cause dementia symptoms, and consulting a specialist can be confusing.

CHAPTER THREE: HOW TO SELECT NATURAL REMEDIES FOR ELDERS

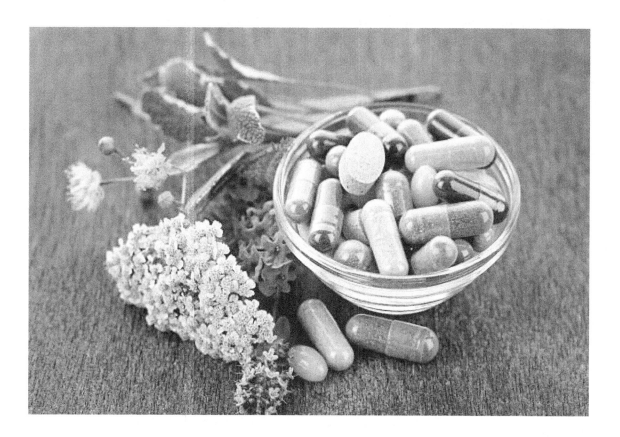

When selecting an herbal medicine, you must exercise caution. Herbal medicines are a form of dietary supplement. They are not pharmaceuticals. As a result, they are more commonly employed to relieve pain rather than to cure it. Herbals are not controlled in the same way that medications are, and they are not rigorously examined. As a result, you must understand why it might not work as advertised. Many individuals believe that treating ailments with plants is "safer" simply because it is natural. While some herbal medicines might benefit you, others can have serious adverse effects. Here are some pointers for selecting herbal medicines for the elderly:

A Trustworthy Brand

Investigate companies that have been producing and distributing high-quality herbal treatments for decades. These businesses are usually reliable because they have been around for a long time. It's never a bad idea to ask questions to figure out what the greatest option is for you.

Look Closely At The Claims

Many herbal medicines have obvious red flags that can be seen right away. You should be careful if the claims seem too wonderful to be true. Keep a close check on the herbal product's description. Is it marketed as a "miracle" tea that can help cure your illness? Is it said that it will be more effective than standard care? It's best to do some research on an herbal treatment before trying it to be sure it's what it claims to be. It's also a good idea to talk to your doctor first so that you may obtain some professional advice on herbal medicine.

Real-Life Stories Are Not Scientific Proof

Many herbal medicines are advertised using "real-life stories" from actual consumers. While these stories may be true to them, you should keep in mind that the effects of herbal medicine may vary from person to person. There is no proof that you will achieve the same outcomes as those described in the stories.

Other Ingredients

Other elements in some herbal medications may be hazardous to your health. This could make the treatment less successful, so it's better to double-check beforehand. Furthermore, herbal medicine may contain components to which you are allergic, causing more harm than benefit to your health. Corn, wheat, soy, and other common allergens should not be included in the product.

Consult Your Healthcare Professional First

Consultation with your doctor is the best method to ensure that the herbal medicine you want to use is safe. This is the best option, especially if you're also taking other medications. The use of an herbal cure and a treatment together could have unfavorable side effects that are more harmful than beneficial. Because your doctor is a trained professional who is familiar with your medical history and problems, he or she will be able to determine what is safe for you to have.

CHAPTER FOUR: RECIPES OF HERBAL REMEDIES FOR ELDERS

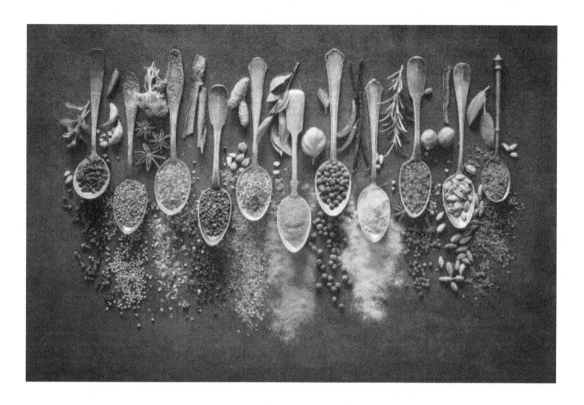

We've offered several recipes in this chapter that use various herbs and spices to assist ease the pain that an elder or loved one may be experiencing. Many elders choose to take a more holistic approach to pain management rather than taking drugs, and they often have items in their homes that they may employ. These recipes are intended to relieve and comfort the user rather than to cure them. The herbal medicines described in this chapter can aid in the treatment of the disorders discussed previously. They are simple to prepare and require only a few ingredients and processes to complete.

Echinacea

Echinacea, also known as "coneflowers," is a flower that can be found all over North America. For centuries, Echinacea Tea has been used to ward off winter infections, proving that it is a powerful immune system stimulant. Neurotransmitters in the brain are triggered by echinacea, which alleviates inflammation in the sinuses and ear tissues. Natural medicines are utilized as both a prophylactic and a curative. It is safe for the elderly and children to use. It not only strengthens the immune system and protects against colds, but it also acts as an antidote to infections that might lead to hearing loss. The echinacea plant's roots, leaves, and blossoms can all be used in natural cures.

Echinacea Tea

This echinacea tea is excellent for easing and reducing the symptoms of a common cold. Echinacea can be used either fresh or dried.

Ingredients:

¼ cup of loose leaf dried echinacea (or ½ cup fresh homegrown echinacea)

1 teaspoon dried lemongrass

1 teaspoon dried mint

8 ounces of boiling water

Directions:

1. Combine all three herbs in a mixing bowl, then add 8 ounces of boiling water.
2. Allow 15 minutes for the mixture to steep.
3. Enjoy plain or with honey.

Echinacea Tincture

One of the most prevalent methods to use echinacea is in tinctures. If you have dried echinacea on hand, this dish is fantastic. Tinctures have a long shelf life and are quite flexible.

Ingredients:

Dried Echinacea

80-proof vodka

Directions:

1. Fill a mason jar halfway with a handful of dried echinacea.
2. Cover the echinacea with alcohol once it has been added.
3. Replace the lid on the jar and shake it vigorously. Keep it for at least a month in a cold, dark place. It should be shaken now and then.
4. The echinacea tincture can now be filtered after 1-3 months. Filter the herbal material from the alcohol with a fine-mesh strainer or cheesecloth.
5. You should be left with a dark, amber-colored liquid that smells strongly of dirt.

Echinacea Flower Infused Honey

This recipe is easy to make if you simply have a few herbal herbs or plants on hand. Fresh echinacea blossoms that have fully flowered are the finest. Using echinacea flower-infused honey to sweeten medicinal drinks is a terrific approach to keep the body healthy.

Ingredients:

Fresh echinacea flower heads
Raw, local honey

Directions:

1. Take a few flower heads from an echinacea plant and cut them off. Allow drying after washing.
2. Once the flower heads have dried, fill a jar halfway with them.
3. Cover the flower head with honey, filling the jar to approximately an inch from the top. Remove any air bubbles by stirring them.
4. Leave the jar covered for about 4 weeks. To ensure a thorough infusion, give the jar a good shake or turn it over.
5. Strain the flowerheads from the honey after 4 weeks and keep the infused honey in a clean jar.

Raw Honey

Raw honey has been used as a folk treatment for centuries and has a wide range of health and medical benefits. Burns, wound healing, swelling, and ulcers inside the mouth, and cough are all popular uses. Honey is high in antioxidants and may aid in the prevention of chronic diseases including cancer and heart disease. Because it naturally includes hydrogen peroxide, an antiseptic, it has antibacterial and antifungal qualities. Raw honey is also utilized in a variety of herbal treatments to help with a variety of ailments.

Honey Thyme Cough Syrup

This mixture is effective in fighting infections and alleviating unpleasant symptoms. Thyme is a potent antibacterial that helps with respiratory infections, while raw honey is fantastic for easing plain.

Ingredients:

2 cups water
3 tablespoons organic fresh or dried thyme
1 cup raw honey

Directions:

1. Place the thyme in a pot of boiling water and steep until the water has cooled completely. It will take about 20 minutes to complete this task.
2. Take the thyme out of the water and stir in the raw honey.
3. Strain the syrup into a clean container and store it for up to two months in the refrigerator.

Honey Eye Drops

Even though there is little clinical research on this natural medicine, many herbal professionals recommend it since it has various benefits for cataract patients. Raw honey has anti-inflammatory and anti-bacterial properties that are good for your overall health and can help prevent cataracts.

Ingredients:

1 cup water

5 teaspoons raw honey

Directions:

1. Bring 1 cup water and 5 teaspoons of raw honey to a boil, continually stirring.
2. Allow for thorough cooling before using the combination.
3. Put the mixture in a sterilized eyedropper and squirt it directly into your eyes to use as an eyewash.

Ginseng

For ages, ginseng has been employed in traditional Chinese medicine. The concentration of active components in American and Asian ginseng differs, as do the effects on the body. American ginseng is thought to have a calming effect, whilst Asian ginseng has an energizing impact. Ginseng has been shown to reduce inflammation, improve brain functions such as memory, behavior, and mood, stimulate the immune system, alleviate COPD symptoms, increase energy, and lower blood sugar levels.

Ginseng Tea

Ginseng Tea might help you feel more energized and ease your nerves. It also aids in the management of cholesterol and blood sugar levels. This tea can significantly boost cognitive health when consumed daily.

Ingredients:

¼ cup American ginseng

6 cups of water

A pinch of salt

Directions:

1. Bring a kettle of water to a boil. Simmer for 5 minutes after adding the ginseng.

2. Season with salt and pepper. Use a strainer to drain the tea and serve at room temperature or chilled.

Ginseng Elixir

This ginseng elixir recipe is used in Chinese medicine for boosting energy, stamina, and longevity. It's a better alternative to caffeine, and it can help you relax, strengthen your immune system, and more.

Ingredients:

8 slices ginseng root (or ¼ cup dried ginseng root)

2 tablespoons ginger, coarsely chopped

2 cinnamon sticks

5 cups water

Almond milk

Raw honey, to sweeten

Directions:

1. Combine ginseng, ginger, cinnamon, and water in a medium pot. Cook for 20 minutes on low heat.

2. Strain out the herbs and sweeten them with almond milk and honey.

3. Serve warm or cold, over ice.

Saffron

Saffron is a vividly colored spice that's high in antioxidants like crocin and crocetin, which are carotenoids. Saffron, interestingly, has shown promise as a natural antidepressant. It has a wide range of plant chemicals that function as antioxidants, as well as cancer-fighting and libido-boosting effects. Saffron may help lower blood sugar levels, enhance vision in adults with age-related macular degeneration (AMD), and improve memory in adults with Alzheimer's disease.

Saffron Milk

Saffron milk, also known as Kesar milk in India, is sweetened milk that has been infused with saffron. Kesar milk is whole milk infused with saffron deliciousness. It is frequently consumed in India because of its health benefits.

Ingredients:

3 cups whole milk

15 saffron strands (a tiny pinch for each cup)

3 teaspoons sugar

Directions:

1. Bring the milk to a boil in a saucepan.
2. Stir in the sugar and strands of saffron. Mix thoroughly.
3. Cook for 3-5 minutes on low heat.
4. Serve hot or warm milk.

Aloe Vera

The antibacterial, antiviral, and antiseptic effects of aloe vera are well-known. This is one of the reasons why it may aid in the healing of wounds and the treatment of skin conditions. Aloe vera has a wide range of therapeutic benefits, particularly as a skin and gum ointment. Aloe vera is sometimes used as a diabetes treatment. This is because it has the potential to increase insulin sensitivity and blood sugar control.

Aloe Vera Gel

Aloe vera gel at home is a simple, straightforward, and low-cost way of extracting gel from aloe vera leaves without having to purchase the product.

Ingredients:

1 big-sized aloe vera leaf

Directions:

1. Take a large aloe vera leaf and trim off the yellow liquid-producing ends.
2. Using a knife, trim the aloe vera leaf's edges and sides. Peeling should be done with caution because it can be somewhat slippery.
3. Make sure only the white area or gel is left after peeling. Using a knife, cut the gel into smaller pieces.
4. Place the gel chunks in a blender and blend until smooth. Add no water to the mix. Simply combine the pieces until a thick gel is formed.
5. Put the gel in a small bottle and keep it in the fridge for at least two weeks.
6. The extracted gel can be applied to the face, skin, or hair externally.

Aloe Vera Juice

Aloe vera juice is simple to make at home, using only two ingredients: an aloe vera leaf and water. Aloe juice offers numerous health advantages. It can aid in digestive and dental health. It also has anti-inflammatory effects, which may aid with arthritic inflammation. It may also help to decrease cholesterol levels and the risk of heart disease.

Ingredients:

½ large aloe vera leaf

1-quart filtered water

2 limes, juiced (optional)

2 tablespoons agave syrup (optional)

Directions:

1. Cut a large aloe vera leaf in half and set it aside. Because the knife is quite slippery, use it with caution.
2. Remove some of the harshness of the aloe gel by rinsing it.
3. In a blender, combine the peeled and rinsed aloe. Combine the water, lime juice, and sweetener in a mixing bowl. Blend until all of the ingredients are thoroughly dissolved.
4. To taste, add additional sweetness or lime. Refrigerate for up to one week or serve immediately over ice.

Turmeric

Turmeric is a spice that may be the most effective nutritional supplement on the market. Turmeric has been shown in numerous high-quality researches to provide significant health advantages for both the body and the brain. Curcumin, the principal active component, is responsible for many of these advantages. Turmeric contains bioactive chemicals that have anti-inflammatory and anti-cancer activities. It's a natural anti-inflammatory substance that may aid in the treatment of arthritis, heart disease, cancer, metabolic syndrome, Alzheimer's disease, and other degenerative diseases. It can increase brain-derived neurotrophic factors (BDNF), which are important for memory and learning. Curcumin has been shown in numerous trials to decrease the progression of lung cancer.

Turmeric Paste

Turmeric paste (also known as turmeric powder paste) is made by heating ground turmeric, oil (coconut oil, ghee, or other neutral oils), water, ground black pepper, and other spices (such as ground cinnamon, cardamom, and ginger) until melted and turned into a paste for use in turmeric milk, smoothies, curries, and other applications. Although turmeric is helpful on its own, we can boost its therapeutic powers by combining it with other healthy components like cinnamon and ginger.

Ingredients:

½ cup ground turmeric spice

1 tablespoon ground cinnamon

1 teaspoon fresh ginger, grated

1 teaspoon black pepper

¼ cup of coconut oil

1 cup water

Maple syrup or raw honey for taste (optional)

Directions:

1. In a small saucepan over medium heat, combine the turmeric spice, grated ginger, ground cinnamon, coconut oil, black pepper, and water.
2. Continue whisking until the oil has completely melted. Be careful not to overheat, as this may cause the turmeric's advantages to be lost.
3. Transfer to a jar and keep it in the fridge once the oil has completely melted and everything has been thoroughly blended.

Turmeric Tea

Turmeric tea is a common way to consume spice. It has a distinct but understated flavor. Turmeric tea is also a terrific way to get the following turmeric health benefits.

Ingredients:

⅓ cup of raw honey

2 ½ teaspoons dried turmeric

Lemon

Freshly ground black pepper

Directions:

1. Combine the turmeric and honey to make a paste.
2. Place a teaspoon of turmeric paste in the bottom of a mug. Fill the mug halfway with hot, but not boiling, water and stir well to dissolve the turmeric paste.
3. Add a decent amount of black pepper and a hefty squeeze of lemon juice.
4. Combine all of the ingredients in a large mixing bowl and stir thoroughly.

Turmeric Golden Milk Elixir

Golden milk is an ancient ayurvedic treatment that helps to improve your immune system and fight colds, coughs, inflammation, joint discomfort, and more.

Ingredients:

1 teaspoon turmeric paste

1 cup milk of choice

1 tablespoon raw honey or maple syrup

¼ teaspoon vanilla extract

Directions:

1. In a small saucepan, combine all of the ingredients. Gently heat and whisk until fully mixed.
2. In a blender, blend until frothy.

Ginger

Ginger is a flowering plant from Southeast Asia. It's one of the world's healthiest (and most flavorful) spices. Ginger has a long history of usage in both conventional and natural medicine. It has been used to assist digestion, relieve nausea, and treat the flu and common cold. It contains potent anti-inflammatory and antioxidant properties that aid in the treatment of a variety of ailments. Nausea, osteoarthritis, and persistent indigestion can all be treated with ginger. It decreases blood sugar levels, which is beneficial for diabetics, as well as cholesterol levels. Ginger also contains a chemical that aids in the prevention of cancer, the prevention of Alzheimer's disease, and the battle against infections.

Ginger Tea

Ginger tea is a soothing beverage to consume, especially if you have a cold or a cough. It's simple to manufacture and everyone has access to it.

Ingredients:

4 thumb-sized fresh ginger roots, peeled and cut

12 cups water

Directions:

1. Peel the ginger with a spoon after washing it.
2. Cut the ginger into matchsticks by cutting it lengthwise.
3. Combine ginger and water in a large pot. Bring the water to a boil.

4. Reduce heat to low and cook for 20 minutes.

5. Strain and pour into a pitcher once it has cooled. The ginger tea can be served hot or cold.

Ginger Tincture

This ginger tincture is a fantastic natural medicine for supporting digestion as well as other problems. It is easily dissolved in a small amount of water. 14 teaspoons is a nice place to start for most adults to explore what you enjoy and how it works for you. 6 to 8 ounces of water, stirred in It can also be used in the kitchen to make juices and smoothies, broths, and soups, yogurt, and more.

Ingredients:

2 cups of 80-proof vodka

½ to ¾ cup of ginger root (dried or fresh, chopped)

Directions:

1. Fill a jar 1/3 full of dried ginger and pour alcohol over the root up to the container's neck.

2. Cover the jar with the lid and shake it a few times. For 4 to 6 weeks, store in a cool, dark place. Shake the jar now and then.

3. Strain and store after 6 weeks.

4. If using fresh ginger root, fill a jar halfway with chopped fresh ginger (no need to peel it beforehand). Pour the alcohol over the root until it reaches the jar's neck.

5. Screw on the lid and give the jar a good shake. For 3 to 4 weeks, store in a cool, dark place. Shake the jar now and then.

6. Strain and store after 4 weeks.

Ginger Ale

Ginger Ale is a tasty and effective natural cure for soothing upset stomachs and fighting colds. The majority of store-bought ginger ales are high in sugar, so you won't receive the true taste or benefits of ginger. As a result, this recipe provides you the authentic taste of ginger ale while also providing several health advantages.

Ingredients:

2-inch piece fresh ginger, juiced or grated

8 ounces of sparkling or carbonated water

½ lemon, juiced or squeezed

1 tablespoon honey

Directions:

1. Juice the ginger and lemon if using a juicer, then combine with the bubbling or carbonated water and honey.

2. If using a blender, grate the ginger and squeeze 12 lemon juice. Combine all of the ingredients in a blender and drain through a fine strainer.

Dandelion

Dandelions are a blooming plant family that can be found all over the world. Dandelion is regarded in traditional herbal medicine for its vast range of therapeutic benefits. They've been used to cure a variety of health conditions for millennia, including cancer, acne, liver disease, and digestive problems. It is high in antioxidants and helps to reduce inflammation. It may help with blood sugar control, cholesterol reduction, and blood pressure reduction. Dandelions can also help to keep the liver healthy and combat cancer. According to certain studies, dandelions may offer antibacterial and antiviral properties, which may help your body fight infection.

Dandelion Syrup

This dandelion syrup is a natural sweetener that is good for you. This syrup is delicious drizzled over pancakes, oats, tea, and more. It's easy to create and has numerous health benefits.

Ingredients:

1 ½ cups dandelion flowers

3 cups water

2 cups cane sugar (or sweetener of choice)

¼ cup raw honey (optional)

½ lemon, juiced (optional)

Directions:

1. Gather some dandelion blooms and put them out on a cloth for an hour. You can also wash the flowers, but this may remove part of the pollen, which is beneficial to your health.

2. Remove the flower's green base and discard it. Because the base is bitter, make sure you remove it completely.

3. Fill a pot with petals and water. Bring to a boil, then reduce to a simmer for 30 seconds to a minute.

4. Turn off the heat and set it aside to cool somewhat. Strain the liquid over a dish the next morning with a fine mesh strainer or cheesecloth.

5. Pour the filtered liquid into a pot with the sugar, honey, and lemon juice, if using. Bring to a boil, then reduce to low heat and cover for 1 hour, or until the liquid has reduced by half.

6. Dip a spoon into the syrup to check the consistency. Remove the pot from the heat when it's done to your liking.

7. Pour the syrup into a glass jar and set it aside to cool to room temperature before keeping it in the refrigerator.

Dandelion Infused Oil

Dandelion oil has a pleasant summer scent and is beneficial to aching muscles and joints. It also has calming effects, which can be paired with lavender to create a relaxing stress-relieving ointment. This dandelion oil is a terrific way to get started with making infused oils from fresh herbs, and it's a great project for the springtime.

Ingredients:

1 cup dandelion flowers, wilted for a day or so
½ cup of carrier oil approximately (you can use a blend of equal parts extra virgin olive oil, coconut oil, and sweet almond oil.)

Directions:

1. Place the withered dandelion blossoms in a container and cover them with your preferred carrier oil. If you want to use coconut oil, you need to melt it first.

2. Store the dandelion oil in a dark area for a week or two, but no longer because it will spoil.

3. Using a fine-mesh strainer or cheesecloth, drain out the blossoms.

Dandelion Salve

Because dandelion flowers offer anti-inflammatory and pain-relieving characteristics, this ointment is suitable for a variety of aches and pains. It is very beneficial to aching and weary muscles and joints. For dry, chapped, and irritated skin, the dandelion salve is also calming and nourishing. It could also be used as a lip balm if your lips are chapped.

Ingredients:

1 cup dandelion infused oil
1-ounce beeswax
1-ounce refined shea butter
12-24 drops essential oils of your choice

Directions:

1. Make a double boiler by placing a small bowl over a saucepan of simmering water with approximately an inch of water.
2. In a small bowl, combine the dandelion oil and beeswax. Heat, stirring occasionally until the beeswax has completely dissolved in the oil.
3. Stir in the shea butter until it is completely dissolved.
4. Add the essential oils and mix well.
5. Carefully pour the salve into small jars or tins and lay aside until totally set.

Capsaicin

Chili peppers contain capsaicin, a substance that gives them their infamous spiciness. Its heat makes it perfect for spicing food while also delivering a variety of therapeutic benefits. Many therapeutic ointments, gels, and patches, especially for illnesses like arthritis, contain capsaicin as the active ingredient. It also has anti-inflammatory properties, making it useful for maintaining heart health and boosting metabolism.

Capsaicin Cream

A popular topical pain treatment that may be created at home is capsaicin cream. It can be used to treat arthritis-related joint pain as well as other unpleasant musculoskeletal diseases. Even deep joints, such as the back, hips, and shoulders, are thought to benefit from it. Capsaicin attaches to nerve receptors and generates a burning, tingling feeling, followed by an analgesic effect or the blockage of pain.

Ingredients:

1 tablespoon organic cayenne pepper
5 tablespoons organic raw coconut oil

Directions:

1. Make a paste using cayenne pepper and coconut oil.
2. Massage the painful region with your fingers.
3. Always wash your hands after using them and keep them away from your eyes, nose, and mouth.

Capsaicin-Infused Water

Vitamin A and vitamin C are among the antioxidants found in capsaicin-infused water. It aids in the reduction of inflammation and is important in the treatment of a variety of chronic illnesses. Drinking this will improve your overall health and speed up your metabolism, which is beneficial if you're trying to lose weight.

Ingredients:

3 cups purified water

½ teaspoon cayenne

1-inch ginger piece, cut into thin slices

½ lemon, cut into slices

1 peach, cut into slices

Directions:

1. Wash and cut all of the ingredients, and then transfer to a pitcher.
2. Combine all ingredients in a large mixing bowl and refrigerate overnight before serving.

Sage

Loss of appetite, gas (flatulence), stomach pain (gastritis), diarrhea, bloating, and heartburn are all symptoms of sage use. It's also used to treat depression, memory loss, and Alzheimer's disease, as well as to reduce excessive sweating and saliva production. Cold sores, gum disease (gingivitis), sore mouth, throat, or tongue, and swollen, uncomfortable nasal passages are all treated with it directly on the skin. For asthma, some people inhale sage.

Sage Herbal Tea

Sage tea is a fragrant beverage brewed from common sage leaves. It has anti-inflammatory and antioxidant components that can aid in the reduction of inflammation and blood sugar levels. It also has wound-healing qualities and may help to protect the skin. Sage tea also contains anti-cancer effects and helps to prevent brain illnesses such as Alzheimer's disease.

Ingredients:

1 tablespoon fresh sage leaves (or 1 teaspoon dried sage)

1 cup water

1 wedge lemon (optional)

Honey, to sweeten (optional)

Directions:

1. Bring a large pot of water to a boil. Remove the pan from the heat and add the sage to the water.
2. Set aside for 3-5 minutes to steep. Strain into a cup and, if preferred, add lemon and honey.

Sage Herbal Salve

Sage Herbal Salve is said to help clear toxins, soothe minor skin irritations, reduce the appearance of blemishes, and treat stretch marks, blisters, and swelling. Its hydrating and conditioning characteristics assist to relieve inflammation and dryness.

Ingredients:

1 cup base oil blend of your choice (you can use coconut oil, olive oil, etc.)
½ cup dried sage
2-4 tablespoons beeswax pastilles
Essential oil of your choice

Directions:

1. Infuse your base oils with dried sage. Strain through a fine-mesh filter when the oil has been sufficiently infused.
2. In a double boiler, pour the infused oil. Warm the beeswax until it has completely melted.
3. Remove the mixture of oil and beeswax from the heat. Mix in your essential oils thoroughly.
4. Pour into individual 2-ounce jars or other jars of equivalent size. Allow it cool completely before covering the container with a lid.

Essential Oils

Aromatherapy, a type of alternative medicine that uses plant extracts to enhance health and well-being, frequently includes essential oils. Essential oils can be inhaled or applied to the skin after being diluted. When ingested, they may heighten your sense of smell or have medical properties.

Tea Tree Oil

Tea tree oil is thought to help with hearing loss and deafness, particularly sensorineural hearing loss, by many people. It contains a lot of terpinen-4-ol, a chemical that kills bacteria when it comes into contact with them. Before using this medicine, you must get medical counsel.

Ingredients:

3 drops tea tree oil
1 tablespoon olive oil
1 teaspoon colloidal vinegar
1 teaspoon apple cider vinegar

Directions:

1. In a small saucepan, combine all of the ingredients and heat over low heat.
2. Pour into a dropper after that.
3. Place the liquid in your ears for five minutes while remaining still.
4. Repeat steps 1–4 four times per day.

Eucalyptus Oil

Eucalyptus trees are native to Australia, but they are currently farmed throughout the world for medical uses. The oval-shaped leaves of eucalyptus trees, which can be transformed into essential oils, have medicinal properties. Eucalyptus oil has been used to cure wounds and infections, as well as to ease coughing. Inhaling steam with added eucalyptus oil can also aid with respiratory issues, and it has diabetes therapy potential. Eucalyptus oil's anti-inflammatory characteristics can help to reduce pain and speed up the healing process, as well as relieve joint discomfort caused by disorders like arthritis.

Ingredients:

30 dried eucalyptus leaves
1 cup coconut oil or olive oil

Directions:

1. Collect some eucalyptus leaves and dry them outside in the sun. After the leaves have dried, put them in a blender and crush them.
2. Fill a jar halfway with crushed leaves.
3. Mix in 1 cup of coconut or olive oil well.
4. Cover the jar and keep it at room temperature for 7-10 days. Every day, give the bottle a good shake.
5. Pour the oil into a pan after 10 days. For 3 minutes, heat the oil over medium heat.
6. Remove it from the oven and set it aside to cool completely. To separate the oil, use a fine-mesh sieve or cheesecloth. Store in a dry, airtight container.

Chamomile Oil

Chamomile is well-known for its anti-inflammatory effects, which make it beneficial to one's health. Chamomile oil can be used to treat eczema, bruising, and even rheumatic pain safely on the skin. Chamomile oil has also been used for generations to treat digestive issues, anxiety, promote calm, and reduce pain from illnesses such as arthritis.

Ingredients:

1 small sterile jar, approx. 100 ml

1 carrier of your choice, sweet almond oil is recommended

Dried chamomile flowers

Directions:

1. Add the dried chamomile flowers to the jar and top it out with the carrier oil. Make sure the oil completely covers the blooms.
2. Cover the container with the lid and place it somewhere where it will receive at least 6 to 8 hours of sunlight per day.
3. Shake the bottle at least once a day. You can filter the oil in about a month.
4. Strain the oil into a clean jar. It's now possible to utilize it straight from the jar.

Lemon Oil

Lemon oil has several advantages. It can help to reduce anxiety, improve digestion, and improve memory. Lemon oil diffused into the air can help elders with dementia overcome emotions of depression and loneliness.

Ingredients:

1 lemon

Cold-pressed olive oil

Directions:

1. Grate the lemon's outside over a small basin. Only the lemon peel can be used to create lemon oil, so ensure there is no fruit pulp or bitter white pith attached.
2. Place grated lemon zest halfway into a small glass bottle. Fill the bottle with olive oil to the top.
3. Place the bottle on a sunny windowsill or in a sunny location.
4. Leave it there for 1-2 weeks, shaking the bottle occasionally.
5. Using a straightener, strain the oil into another glass jar.

CONCLUSION

Herbs are all around us, yet we don't always recognize or appreciate them. Dandelions, for example, are one of several herbs that have numerous health advantages. Many people think of dandelions as a bothersome weed that needs to be mowed, yet they are regarded as a "super herb" because of their numerous health advantages. Similarly, there are a variety of spices with numerous health benefits that can be found in our kitchens and that we are unaware of. Here are a few last pointers to remember before you go on a new life of using natural medicines to improve your health:

It is important to note that natural therapies are not cures. They are simply used to alleviate pain, enhance immune systems, and other things. They are unable to cure a specific medical condition that may necessitate more aggressive therapies, such as surgery. It is critical to seek medical advice before using any natural remedy, since it may interact poorly with your body and so become more hazardous. This is particularly true if you're also using other drugs or herbal supplements. Combining these medications could result in life-threatening consequences.

If you want to incorporate herbs and spices into your wellness routine, consider why you want to do so. Is it beneficial to your general well-being? Do you have a specific concern that you'd like to discuss? Some herbs and spices are gentle enough to be used daily and are beneficial to one's overall health. Herbs like chamomile, echinacea, ginger, and others are among them. If you want to address a specific condition, however, you should seek professional help. You'll obtain an appropriate dosage that's safe, effective, and tailored to your specific needs this way. This could include an herbal formula with precise ratios of a variety of herbs to maximize their effectiveness. The herbs used for overall well being and specific illnesses may be the same, but the frequency, amount, or type of extract utilized differs. It's easy to become perplexed, which is why, if you're suffering from a certain ailment, you should seek medical advice.

When you're ready to buy herbs and spices for your natural treatments, think about the quality and potency of the herb or spice, how it should be prepared, if it's ethically and sustainably sourced, and what foods, medications, or behaviors might aid or hinder the effects. Most importantly, you should determine whether a herb or spice is suitable for you, your body, and your unique health requirements.

When it comes to natural treatments, there are numerous ways to use or prepare them. This book includes many recipes to aid with your preparation. Herbs and spices can be converted into a variety of products, including infusions, tinctures, teas, balms, and salves. The method you choose will be determined by what you want to do with it, how it will be stored, and how long you want it to last.

Because the US Food and Drug Administration (FDA) does not regulate herbs and supplements, many of the goods on the market aren't evaluated for quality, potency, or contamination. According to a 2019 study, nearly half of the herbal products examined had DNA, chemical composition, or both contamination concerns. Dust, pollens, insects, rodents, parasites, germs, fungi and mold, poisons, pesticides, poisonous heavy metals, prescription medications, and filters are all examples of contaminants. It is up to the consumer to conduct their research in the absence of rules. One approach to assure you're getting top-notch quality is to buy herbs from a respected, competent practitioner.

When you're stuck, many herbal specialists can share their knowledge and assist you. Herbal medicine certifications come in a variety of forms. Because herbal guidance is not a licensed profession, some persons may provide it with little or no training. Others have completed their schoolings, such as master's degrees and doctorates in herbal medicine, and are licensed in their respective states. Consider seeing a naturopathic doctor (ND) or a qualified acupuncturist if you prefer to visit a licensed professional. The appointments are even covered by some insurance companies.

Natural remedy use is a complicated science that draws on a wide range of traditions, civilizations, and worldviews. There is no such thing as a one-size-fits-all solution. The safest and most effective method to utilize herbs to support your health and wellness is to work with a competent practitioner. Herbal medicine can be a powerful spoke on the wheel of total health with a little research and advice from trained professionals.

Made in the USA
Las Vegas, NV
06 October 2021